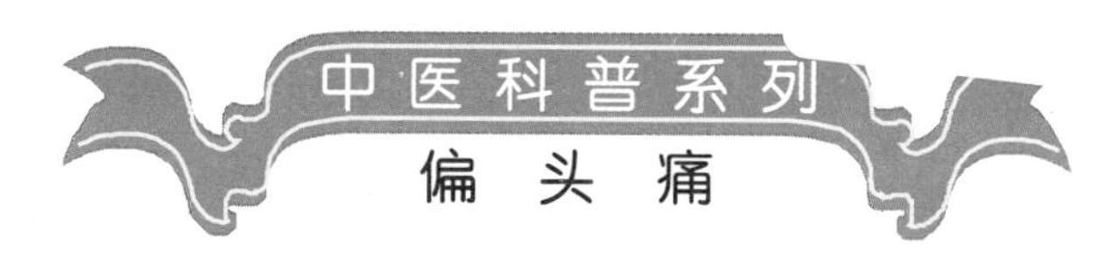

Migraines

Help From Chinese Medicine

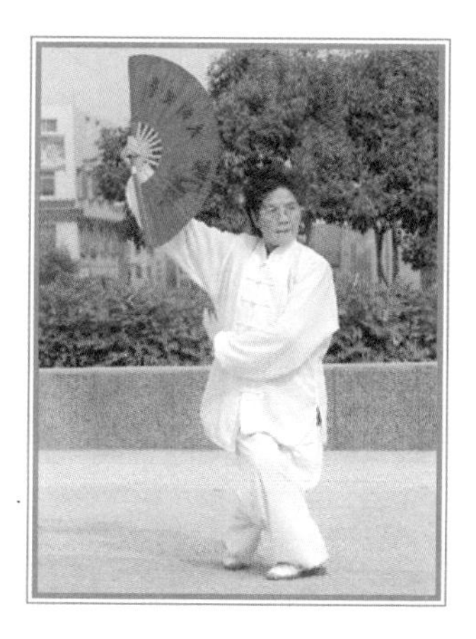

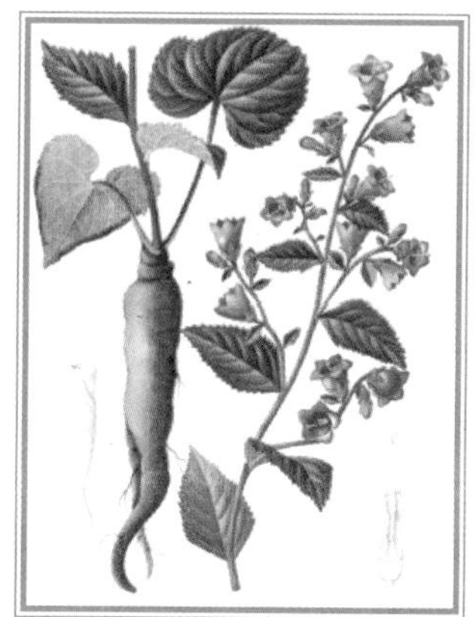

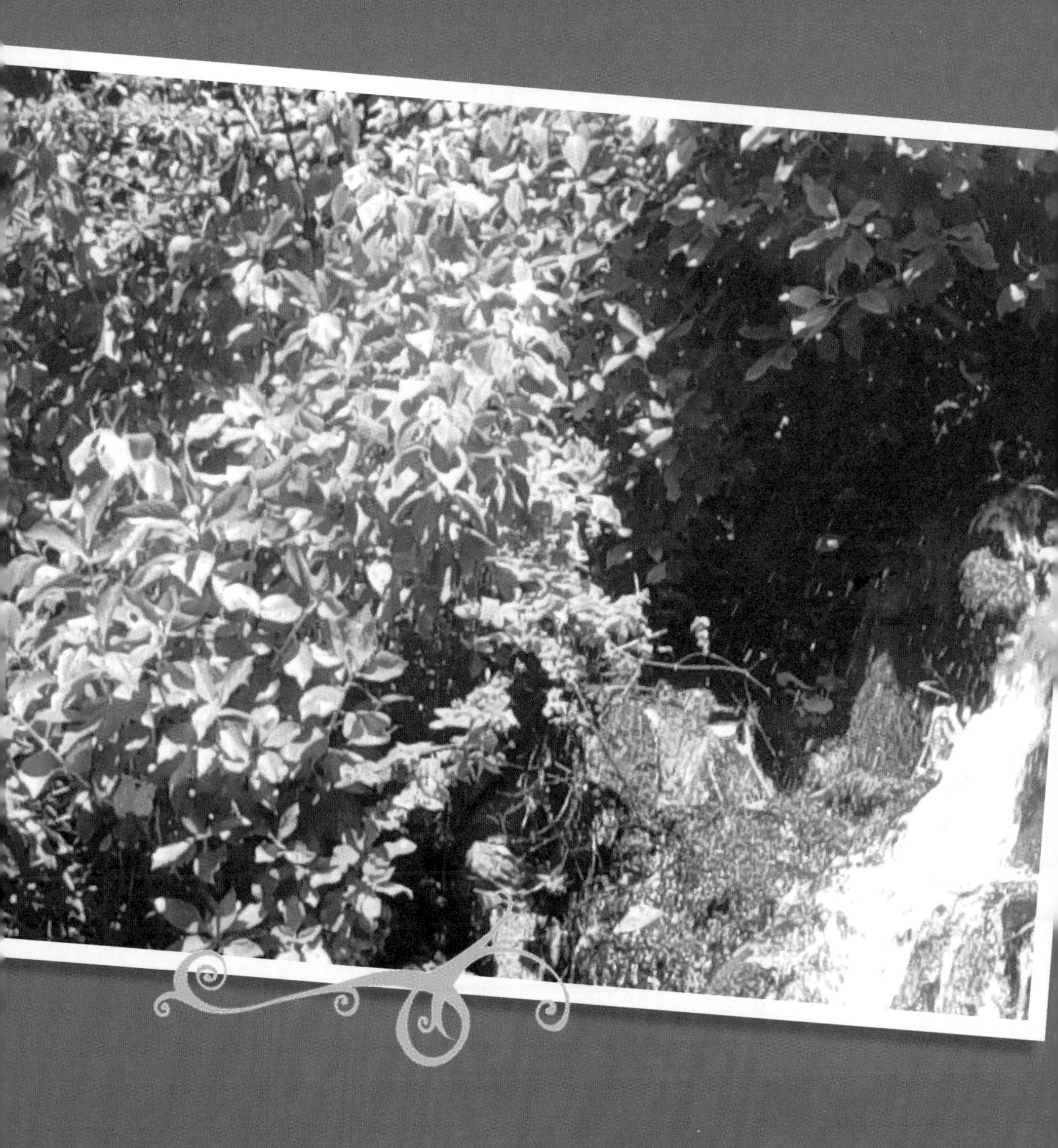

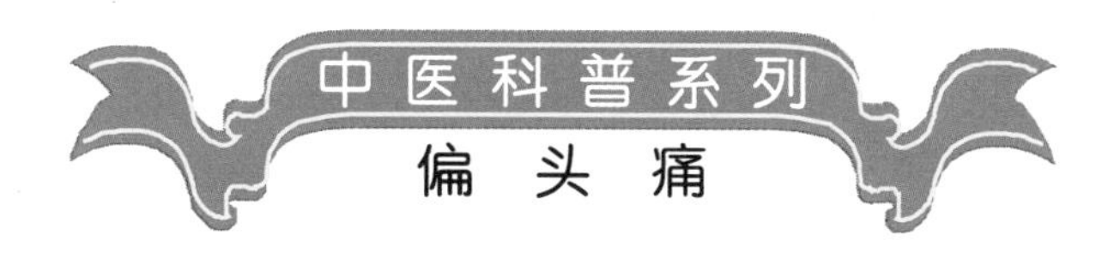

Migraines

Help From Chinese Medicine

Wang Lei, Ph.D. TCM
Carl Stimson, L.Ac.

Edited by John Renna

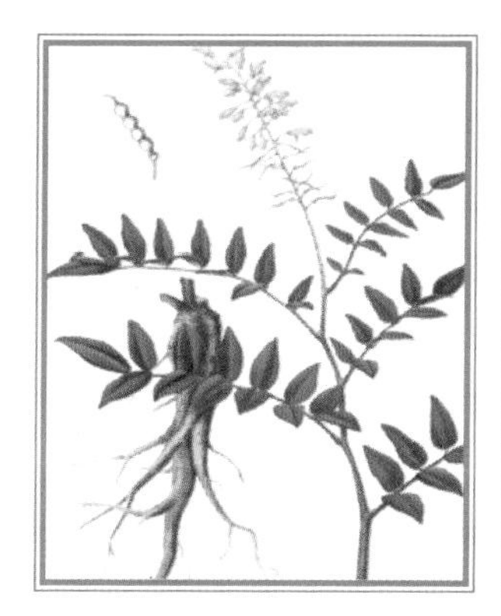
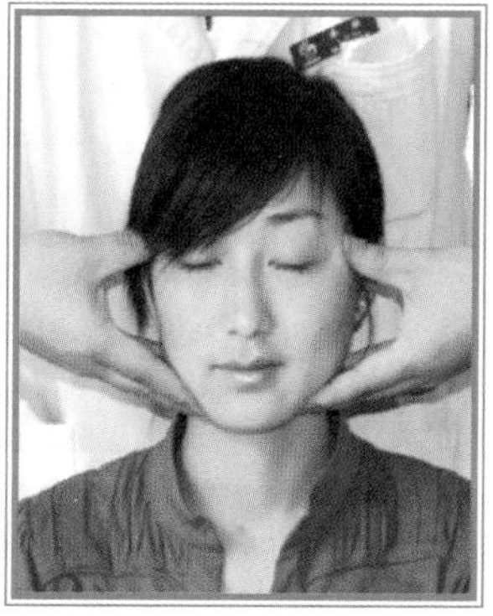

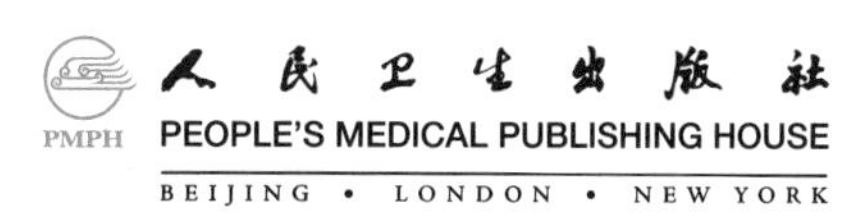

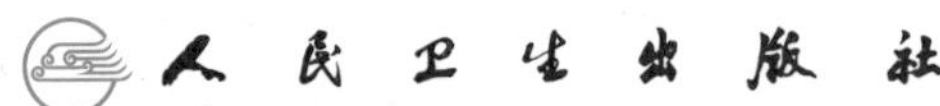

Website: http://www.pmph.com

Book Title: Migraines - Help From Chinese Medicine
中医科普系列——偏头痛

Contact address: Bldg 3, 3 Qu, Fangqunyuan, Fangzhuang, Beijing 100078, P.R. China, phone/fax: 8610 6769 1034, E-mail: pmph@pmph.com

For text and trade sales, as well as review copy enquiries, please contact PMPH at pmphsales@gmail.com

First published: **2008**
ISBN: 978-7-117-10505-7/R·10506

Cataloguing in Publication Data:
A catalog record for this book is available from the CIP-Database China.

Printed in The People' s Republic of China

Foreword

Migraine headaches are a kind of recurrent pulsitile, or throbbing, headache which affect significantly more patients than other types of headache. Before the onset of the headache, there often will be an "aura" such as flashing light, blurred vision, or body numbness. A few minutes to an hour later, throbbing pain located on either side of the head occurs, and often the discomfort increases to the point of nausea or vomiting. For some, a quiet dark environment or sleep is essential to relieve the pain. There may be neurological or psychological dysfunction prior to its onset. Over time, the disease can increase in both intensity and frequency. According to one research report, migraine headache patients are more likely to develop focal brain injuries which can lead to stroke. The more frequent the onset of migraine, the larger the injured area[1].

The causes and symptoms of migraine headaches are diverse. The attacks may frequently recur, forcing some patients to pay continual and significant medical expenses. The purpose of most pharmaceutical medicines is to treat the symptoms, then stop further advancement of the headache. Migraines fall into two categories: organic and non-organic. An organic migraine comes from a distinctly identifiable physical problem such as a lesion or tumor, and in these cases, surgery may be the best treatment option. But for non-organic migraines, if the causes are first identified then removed or avoided, they can be treated without severe methods such as surgery. Currently, most chemical medicines act to relieve pain, but many patients who take prescription medicines for a long time become dependent or create a tolerance to the drug(s), which at the very least, can impact therapeutic efficacy later.

Most patients with migraines develop other psychological burdens that can disrupt daily life and these secondary symptoms can form a vicious cycle of imbalance. For example, a migraine may lead to insomnia; poor sleep can lead to weakness, mental exhaustion or increased muscle tension and these in turn may cause more frequent headaches. Because of the debilitating nature of migraines, a person may also suffer socially and professionally, having to leave work during an attack, call in sick or cancel social engagements. Thus discomfort and problems stemming from the root may branch out to cause other lasting health problems.

Chinese Medicine has long recognized, understood, and treated headaches. For thousands of years its methods have been widely used and practiced, spreading in recent years to nearly every country in the world.

Chinese medicine is best characterized by its naturalistic philosophy of healing the body, which serves to guide all treatments. This philosophy understands the complex workings of the natural world and uses these principles to adjust imbalances that are the source of disease. Far more than simply a traditional or folk healing practice, Chinese medicine aims to improve the body's overall function, slow the progress of disease, and improve the quality of life. In addition, Chinese medicine can be combined with biomedical treatment in order to provide individual therapeutic results.

This book has been written to introduce patients to the treatment of migraines with Chinese medicine. The intention is to provide another horizon for those who are open-minded and willing to see the world differently. It seems you are one of them since you opened this book.

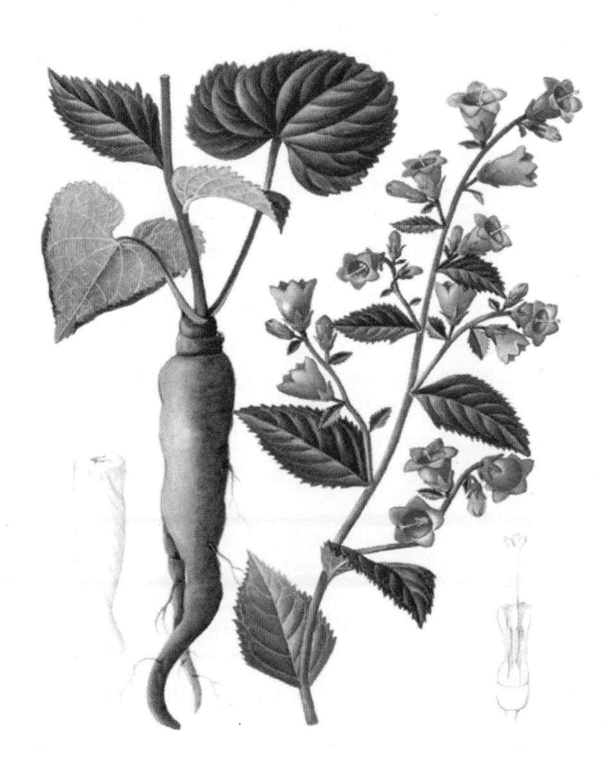

Adenophora

Guide to the book

This book is designed to accomplish two things for you.

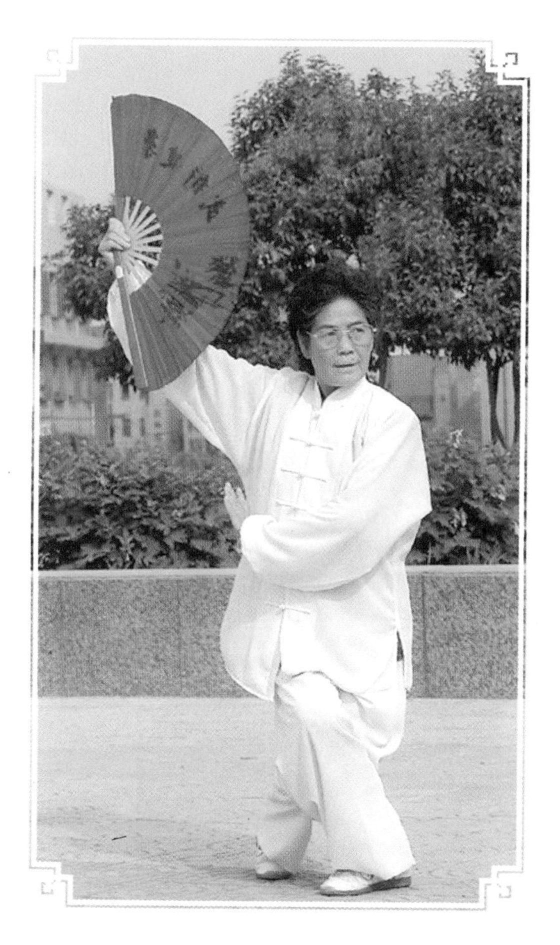

Explain

You may be considering treatment for migraines with Chinese medicine but wonder what treatment will be like. Or, you may have already begun treatment and want to know more about the theories and methods used and participate more fully in the changes happening to you. If you find yourself in one of these situations, then this is the right book for you. It will help you better understand what Chinese medicine is, how it can help, and what is involved in treatment. Several basic theories will be introduced and the methods used by practitioners around the world will be explained in detail. Explanations of commonly known techniques such as acupuncture and herbal medicine, as well as lesser known modalities like moxa and tui na (massage), will help clear up questions or misconceptions as well as prepare you for treatment. And lastly, where available, excerpts from recent biomedical research and clinical trials are included to inspire confidence in the ancient theories and methods.

Guide

The second purpose of this book is to provide you with a resource that can be used to help implement lifestyle changes that will alleviate symptoms as well as increase general health and prevent future illness. Included are helpful information on eating habits, exercise programs, and a variety of at-home treatments that are both easy and affordable. From experience, doctors of Chinese medicine know that with proper treatment, the amount and intensity of biomedical intervention necessary can be reduced or even eliminated. It is our hope that with this book as a guide, all kinds of medical intervention can be reduced so that your time, energy, and money can be better spent doing the things you love.

While there is a lot of valuable information in the following chapters, this book is not intended to substitute for the care of a trained professional. Making a proper diagnosis and prescribing effective treatments are skills that take years to master, especially in complex problems such as migraine headaches. Chinese medicine is a highly individualized system and the help of a proper guide, especially in the beginning stages of treatment, is essential. For suggestions on how to find a qualified practitioner of Chinese medicine, please see the appendix.

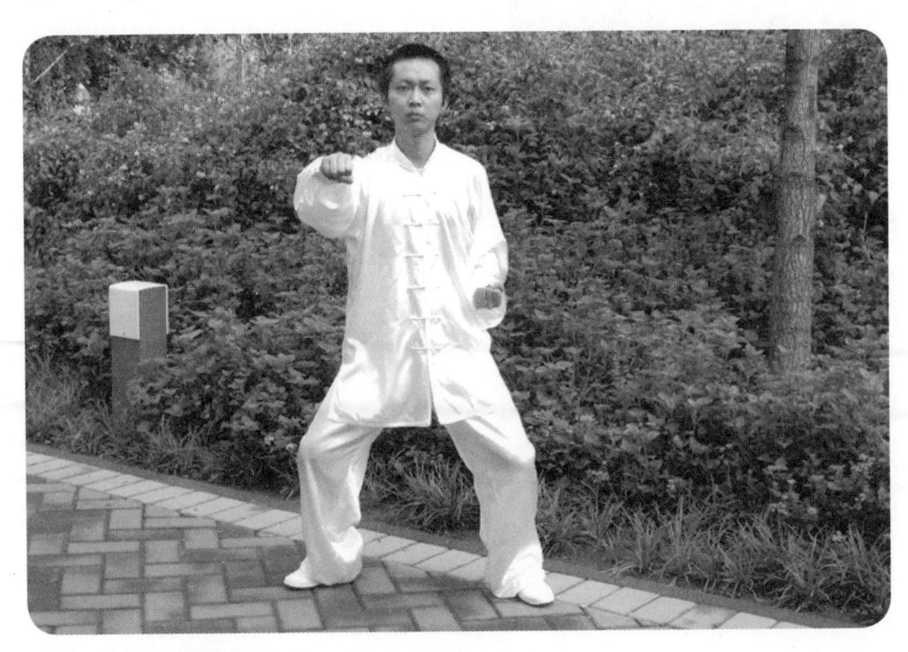

Table of Contents

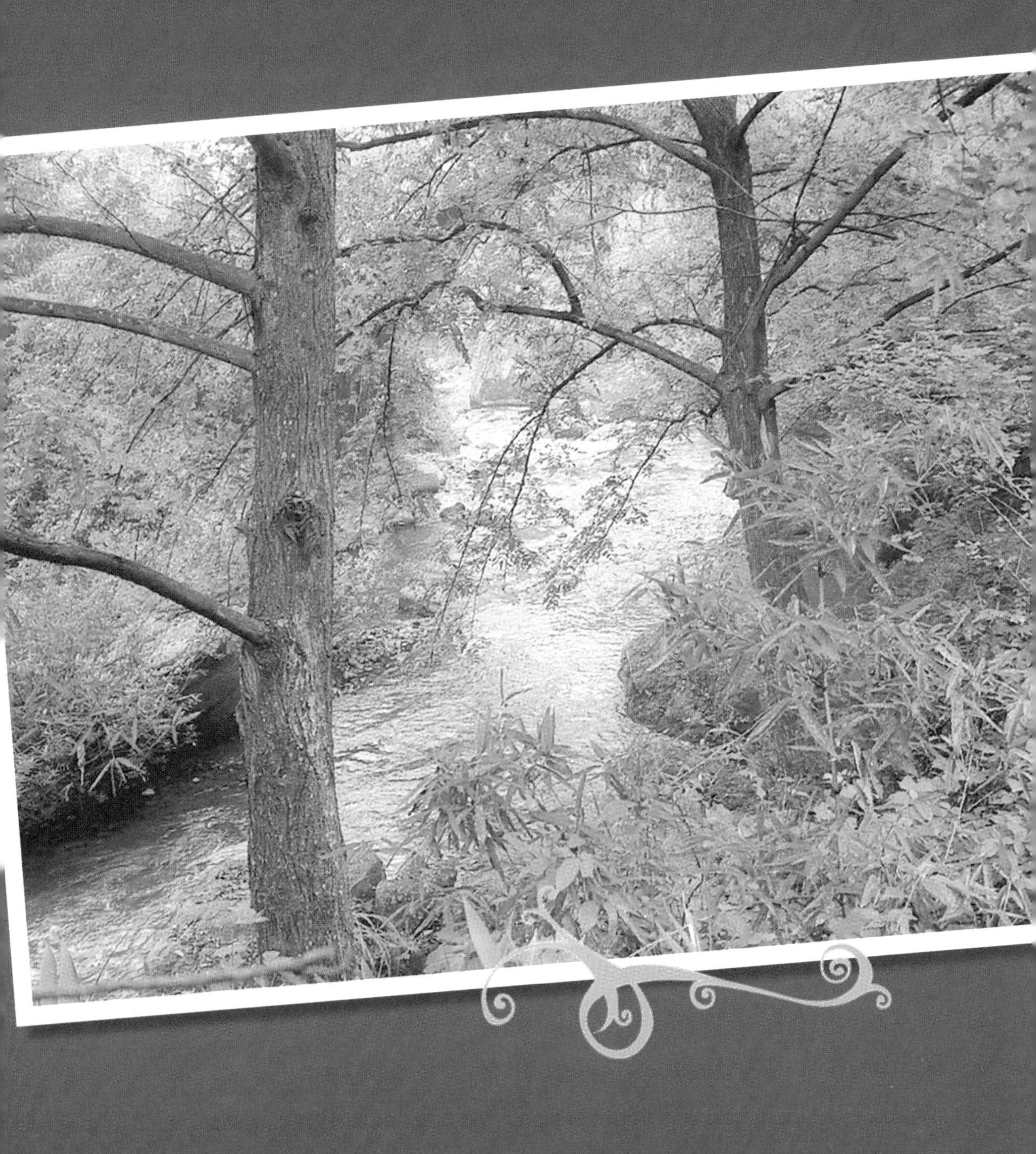

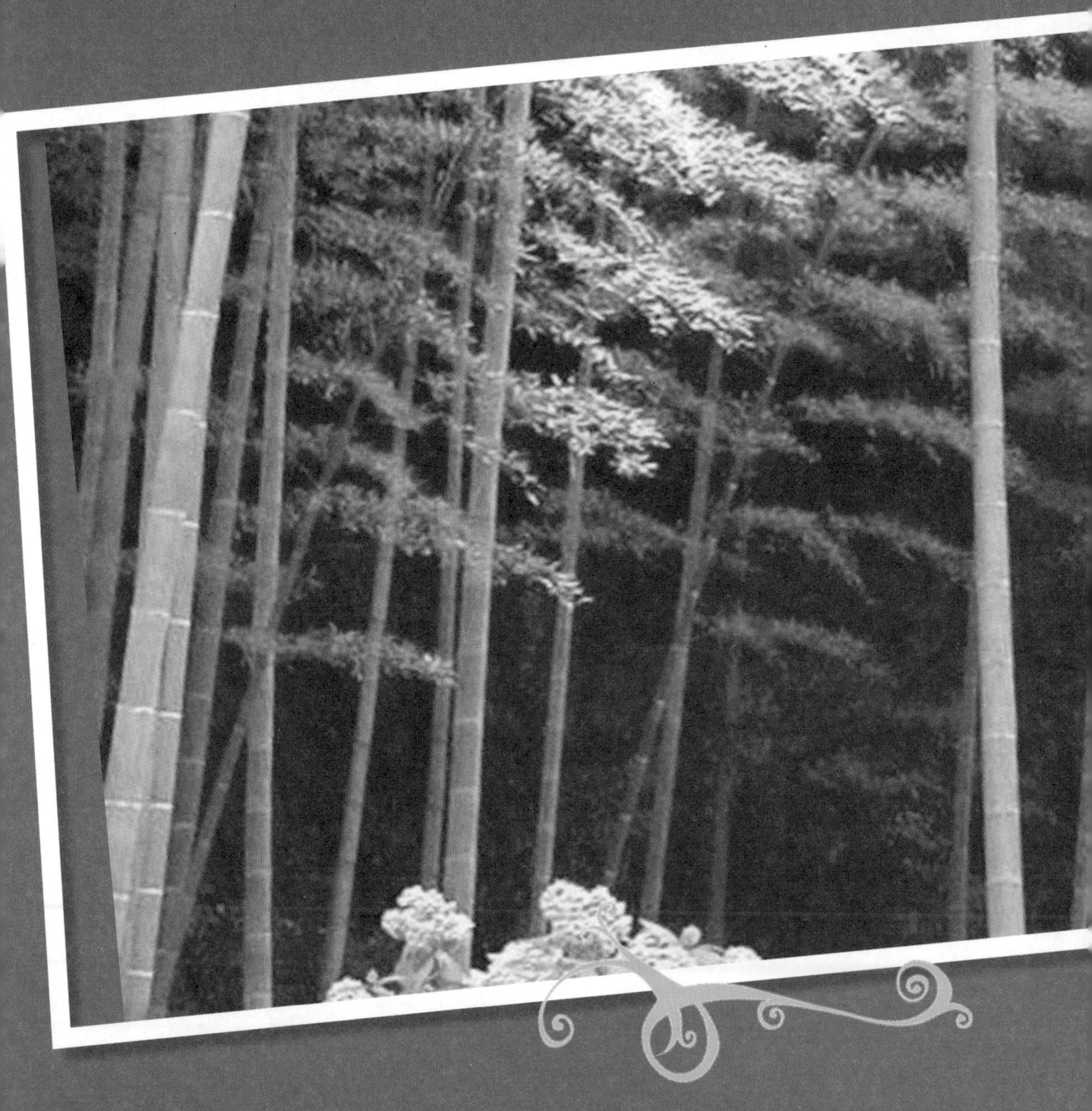

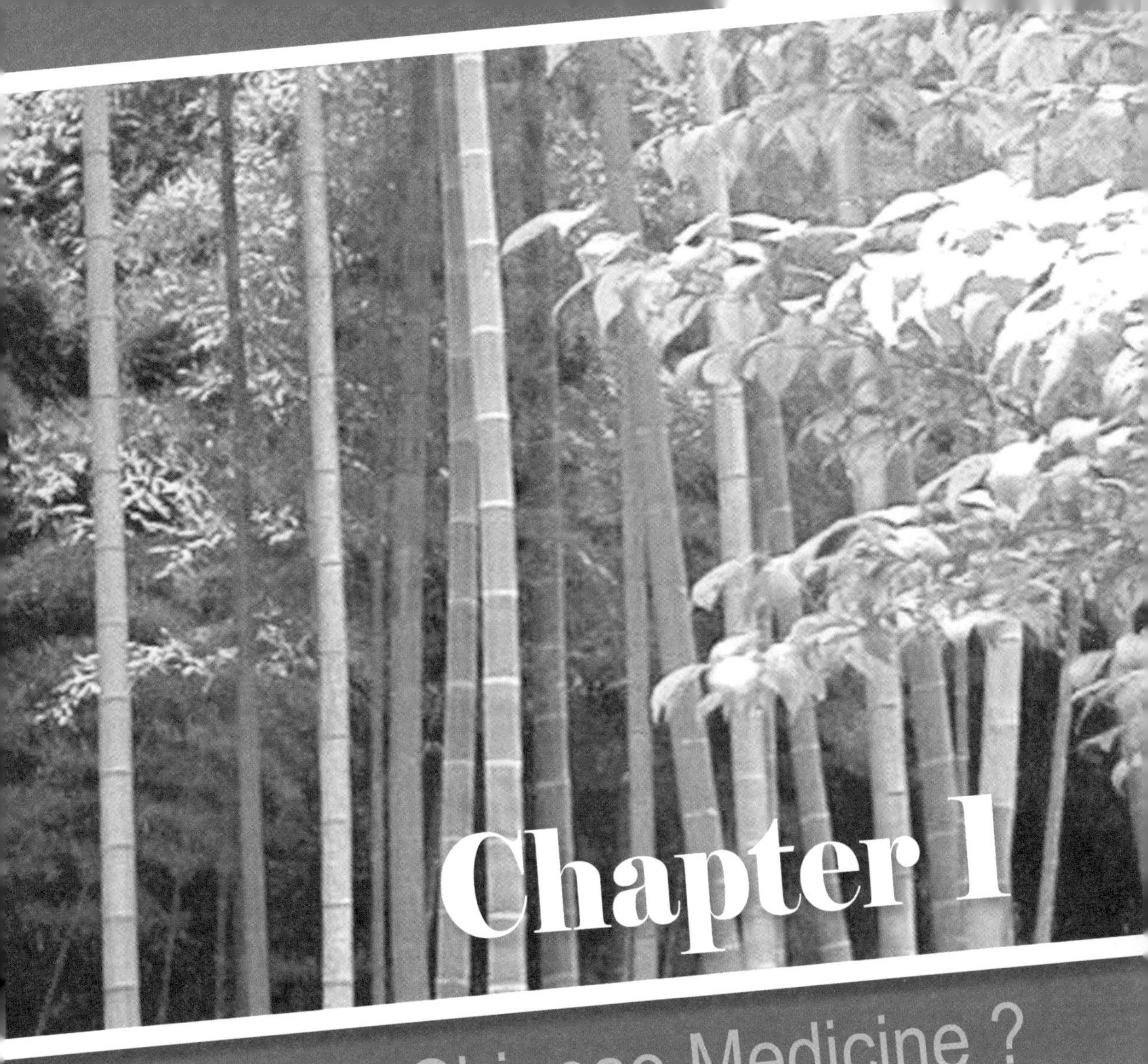

Chapter 1

Why Chinese Medicine ?

Chinese Medicine Worldwide

In China, traditional medicine and biomedicine coexist. What they study and who they serve are the same. Each is an effective weapon against disease, and each has advantages and disadvantages. During their evolution they are sure to influence each other as well as compensate for each other's shortcomings. As modern medicine develops, the model shifts from a pure biomedical framework to a biomedical-psychological-sociological one. The living body is recognized as a diverse material system. The idea of treating the human body as a whole will help the development of medicine in the modern world. We hope in the near future, Chinese medicine and biomedicine will be able to fuse to form a new medical system. Chinese medicine is destined to benefit the health of the whole world.

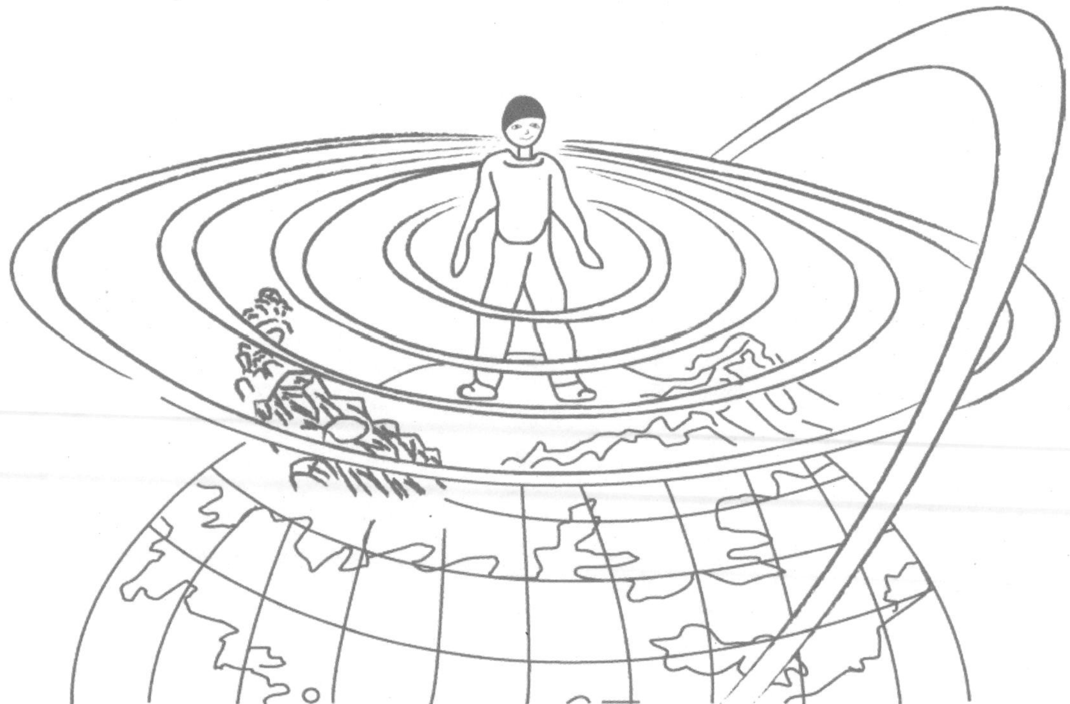

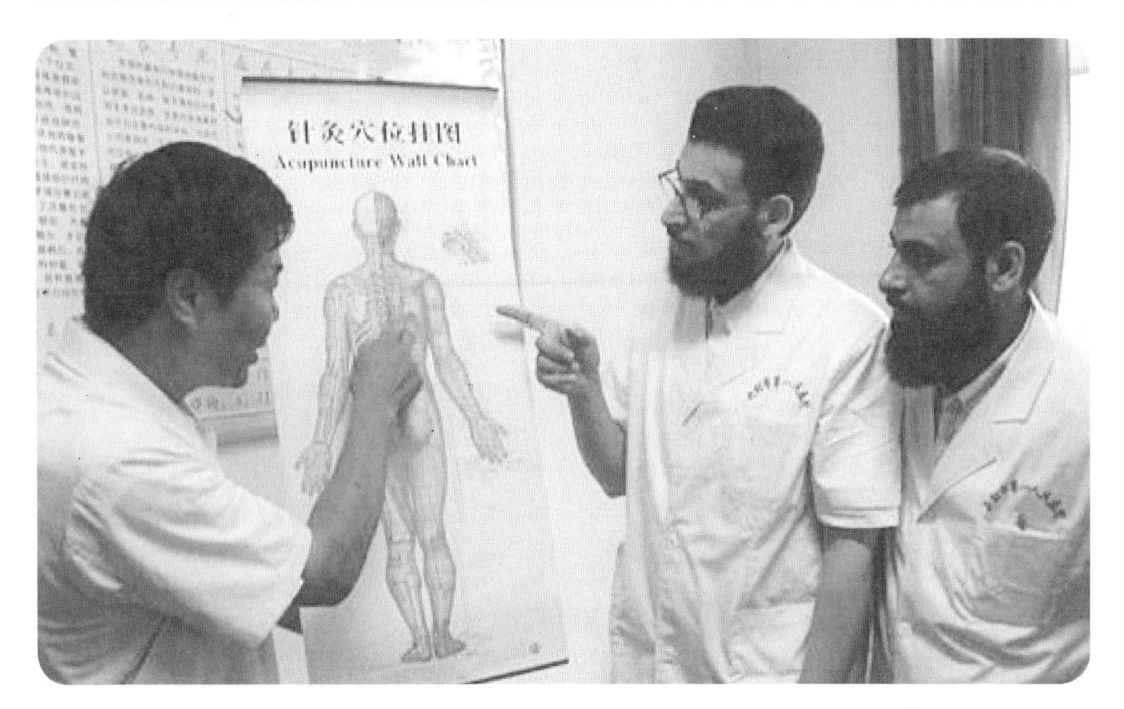

According to incomplete statistics, Chinese medicine has spread to more than 140 countries and regions of the world. Outside of China there are thousands of institutions of Chinese medicine and acupuncture, and more than 20,000 doctors practice Chinese herbalism, while 100,000 practice acupuncture. Thousands of foreign students flood into China to study Chinese medicine in order to discover the secret behind the profound skills of acupuncture, massage, herbal medicine, and health cultivation. At the same time, many countries, including the United States, Canada, Australia, New Zealand and England offer degrees in Chinese medicine.

According to German healthcare statistics, Chinese medicine, especially acupuncture, has won the hearts of the German public with more than 2,000,000 people having sought acupuncture treatments. In Germany 50,000 doctors, one sixth of all physicians, are trained in Chinese medicine. According to the ratio of doctors practicing acupuncture to the population at large, there are more Chinese medicine doctors in Germany per-capita than in China. One opinion poll found 70% of patients surveyed are willing to accept acupuncture treatment, while 31% percent had already used Chinese medicine, and most of the respondents were satisfied with the results of treatment.

In August 2003 the government of British Colombia, Canada, issued senior Chinese medicine doctoral certificates to over two hundred practitioners, and more than six hundred certificates were issued registering standard Chinese medicine doctors, herbal medicine pharmacists and acupuncturists. These are the first group of Chinese medicine doctors officially recognized by the local government and healthcare administration of Canada, and also of North America. Chinese medicine prevails in Canada, not only because of its special curative effect, but also due to its low cost which is far below that of biomedicine. The adoption of Chinese medicine is a good choice for the Canadian government to curb its healthcare financial burden.

Side-effects of pharmacological medicine drive many Swiss to Chinese medical treatments. They understand that Chinese medical theory comes from the principles of balance in nature and that it is, "soft, painless and safe." Many Swiss doctors trust Chinese medicine, especially for chronic pain, allergies and depression. According to statistics there, 700 doctors in Switzerland now practice Chinese medicine.

Chinese medicine has grown quickly in the United Kingdom as well. Herbal pharmacies began expanding out from Chinatown in the mid 1980's. At present, we find more than 3,000 Chinese medicine clinics and drugstores spread all over England, Scotland, Ireland and Wales, with four hundred alone in the greater London area. Many patients not satisfied with their biomedical treatments switched to Chinese medicine. This medicine has also won recognition among the two hundred registered alternative medical practitioners in the U.K. and has become the most popular form of complementary medicine. The British government is trying to further legitimize Chinese medicine through legislation.

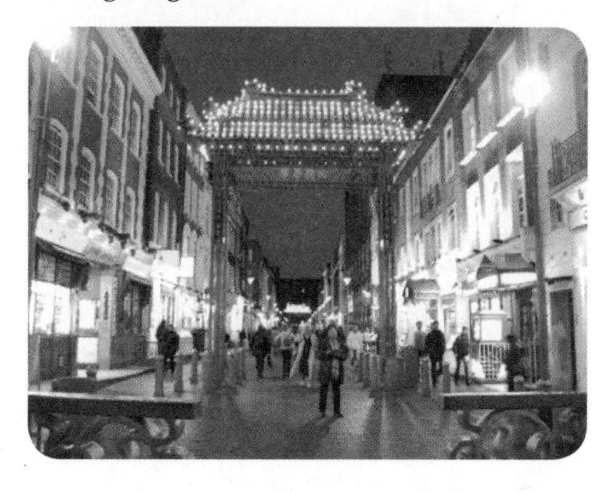

Traditional Chinese medicine is regarded as an effective and inexpensive healthcare option by the National Institute of Health in the United States and widely used among Americans. The population has gradually accepted Chinese medicine since its origin there in 1971. Recent opinion polls show that Chinese medicine is gaining in popularity among people of all ages. Increasing numbers of medical doctors suggest their patients utilize alternative medicine, including Chinese medicine, especially for cancer. This trend is reflected in increased insurance coverage, including Medicare coverage in the state of California. As demand for alternative medicine grows, research and education development also grow. Non-biomedical medicines such as Chinese medicine are included in the curriculum of more than forty biomedical medical schools in the United States, including Harvard Medical School. Meanwhile, Chinese medicine has been successful in helping to treat countless diseases including dermatitis, hepatitis, AIDS, and psychological disease in the U.S.

The World Health Organization (WHO) compiled Chinese medicine clinical guidelines in 2005. These include standardization for basic medical terminology and acupuncture points. Additional projects have already begun that include ophthalmology and cancer therapies using Chinese medicine. Representatives from the WHO reported at conferences in China that the final product will contain guidelines on treating twenty-seven diseases using Chinese medicine[2].

From the introduction above we can see how quickly Chinese medicine has developed and spread throughout the world. With this positive basis we believe Chinese medicine is destined to help relieve people's suffering and treat disease all around the globe in the near future.

This explosion of popularity has taken place over only the past few decades. Techniques that have been used in Asia for

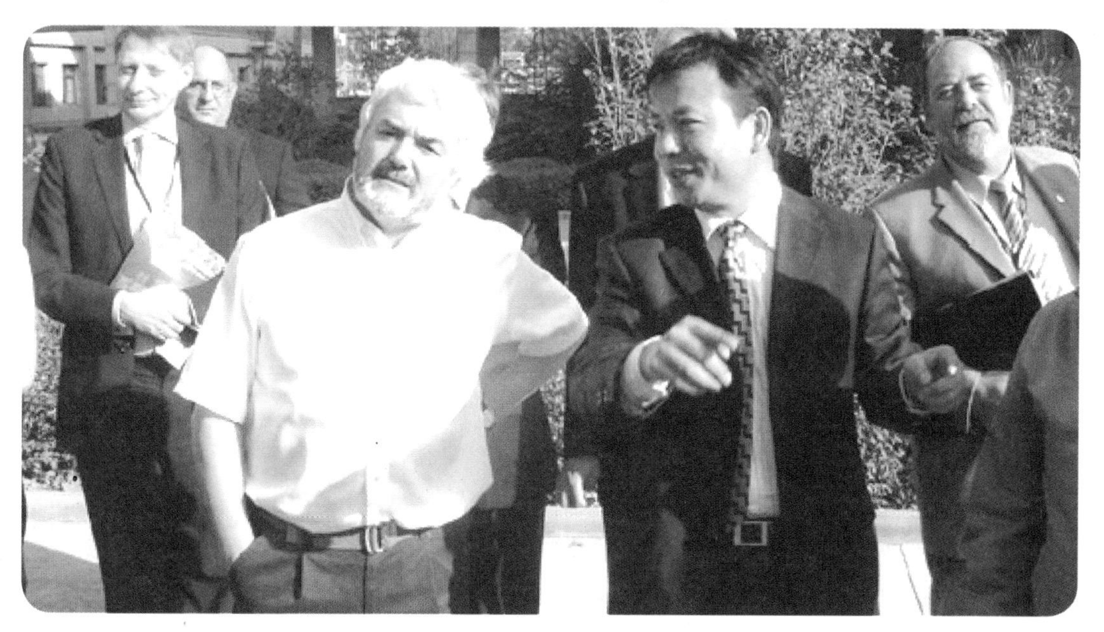

thousands of years have finally found their way to the West and are being heartily embraced. Acupuncture, tai ji, and yin-yang theory seem to be everywhere recently. The biomedical community has taken notice, and government sponsored research on Chinese medicine and other natural medicines now reach nearly $300 million dollars every year in the USA[3]. The public is also interested and acupuncture appears in places from The Oprah Winfrey Show to hip-hop lyrics.

Chinese medicine developed over centuries of combat with disease. It has survived for thousands of years, showing a strong vitality. Looking at the progress and widespread use of this medicine today, it is obvious that its survival depended on its ability to integrate with the leading sciences of the time. This included sciences such as astronomy, mathematics and philosophy in ancient times, and biology and chemistry in the present era. For Chinese medicine to progress further and bring even greater benefit to the world, it must be studied and developed with all available scientific methods.

Despite the temptation and tendency to, Chinese medicine can not be compared across the board with biomedicine. Before comparisons are made, those making the comparisons should be familiar with each system. While evaluation of the efficacy of Chinese medicine needs to be in line with modern research standards, the unique characteristics of diagnosis and treatment in Chinese medicine make it difficult to fit it into research methods that have been tailored for biomedical study. Furthermore, there are fundamental differences between Chinese medicine and biomedicine that lie outside the realm of lab tests and clinical trials. The two systems are different in terms of their philosophy, principles, and approach to treatment. As you read this book, we hope you will begin

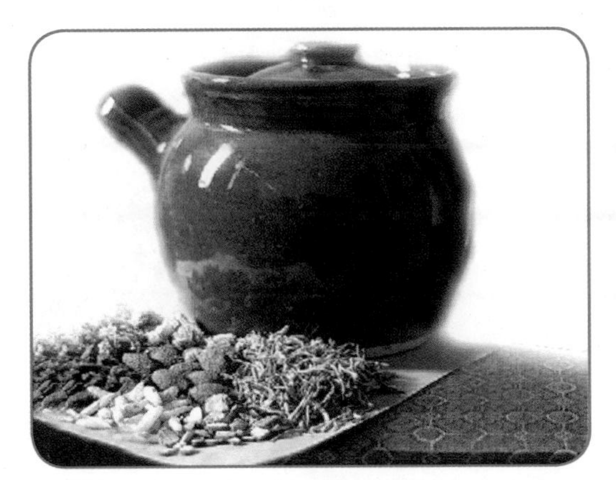

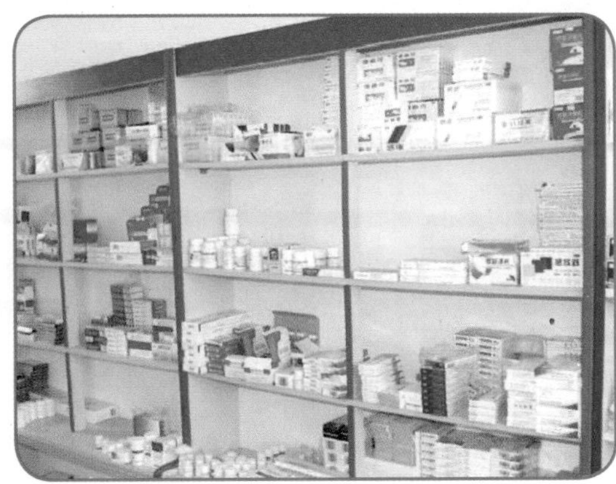

to understand the power and subtlety the Chinese system has to offer.

Chinese medicine can offer a transformational experience for those who suffer from migraine headaches or any other disease. Treatment goals go beyond eliminating and stopping the headache. It is about recovering your natural ability to heal and relieving discomforts which may not go away even if your body is free of the migraine. The ultimate goal is to improve your quality of life, maximize your sense of well-being, eliminate or delay complications, and achieve a longer and happier life.

While biomedical treatment thrives in emergency rooms and during surgery, it often loses its power when faced with the many chronic diseases plaguing developed societies, especially diseases like heart disease, stroke, cancer, diabetes, and lung disorders, which are now labeled the world's leading killers in industrialized nations by the WHO. With migraines specifically, the problem lies primarily in a lack of a comprehensive treatment plan and lifestyle management program. Due to the increasing dissatisfaction of patients with their treatment regimens, one has to wonder if biomedicine is really capable of comprehensive treatment.

Administering pharmaceutical drugs that substitute for a weakened bodily function or artificially replace an insufficient substance can make a patient's laboratory results look better and may even make the patient feel better, but often come with uncomfortable side-effects and lead to difficult complications over time. Many drugs for migraines are intended to be taken for life. Therapies such as these are clearly not aimed at restoring the body's own ability to maintain health.

The examples that follow show several different migraine treatment strategies for a biomedical physician. In the clinic a doctor will generally treat migraines with one or more pain-killing drugs, and the patient may also take that medication with caffeine for better results. Butalbital, a barbiturate, is often used with a pain-killer and caffeine in a combination commonly labeled Fioricet. Butalbital may be used safely and effectively with Paracetamol and Dichloralphenazone, a sedative hypnotic. Another method for treating acute migraine attacks applies a pain-killer plus an antiemetic (to prevent vomiting) and then an anti-anxiety medication. Additionally, stronger acting pain-killers including Dextropropoxyphene, Pethidine, Morphine and Oxycodone, may be prescribed. Still other drugs are used for migraine prevention: beta-adrenergic blocking agents, thymoleptics, calcium channel antagonists, botox scalp injection, 5 - HT antagonists such as cyproheptadine or methysergide, and anticonvulsants are all possible options for a patient suffering from migraines. All of the above medications can cause side-effects during their course of use[4-10].

Most pain-killers carry a risk for dependence and side-effects such as dizziness, tingling or numbness, abdominal spasms, chest distress, or coronary artery spasms. Beta-blocking agents create behavioral side-effects such as sleepiness and other sleep disorders, lassitude, mental depression, forgetfulness and possibly even hallucinations. Frequent physical side-effects of beta-blocking agents include digestive problems and less frequently seen problems that include postural hypotension, a slow heartbeat, and impotence. Beta-blockers can worsen congestive heart failure, Raynaud's syndrome, and diabetes. Thymoleptics can cause dry mouth and increased appetite. Side-effects of calcium channel blockers include dizziness, headache, mental depression, fremitus, digestive complaints, peripheral edema, postural hypotension and a rapid heartbeat.

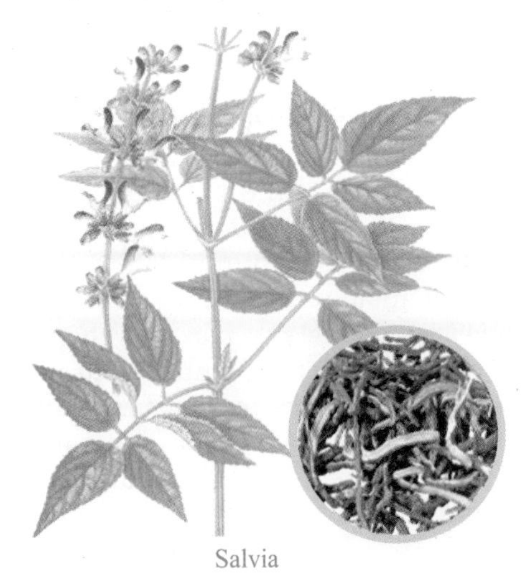
Salvia

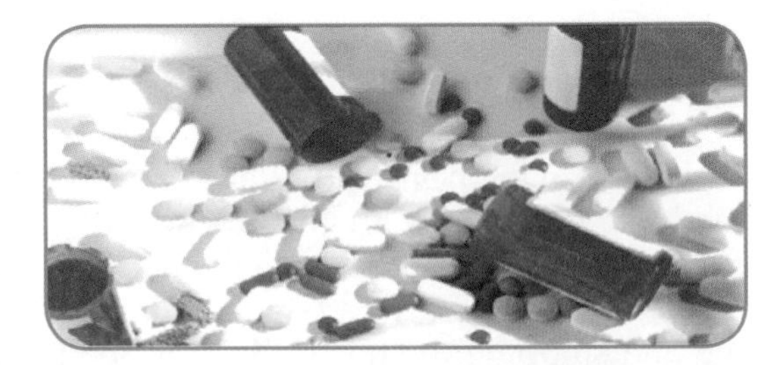

This is not meant to say that biomedicine does not have its merits. Many drugs produced today do wonderful things with very few side-effects, especially if their dosage is low or the administration period short. Indeed, all patients presently under the care of a biomedical doctor should continue their biomedical treatment, even while getting treatment with Chinese medicine, unless specifically instructed not to by either practitioner. When progress is made, the reduction or elimination of biomedical treatment should be done under a doctor's supervision. However, not attempting to restore the body's innate ability to maintain itself is contrary to the fundamental principles behind Chinese medicine. Great importance is given to the concept behind the cliché, "Use it or lose it." The important analogy here is that the use of drugs that substitute for a function or substance will help relieve symptoms in the short term, but will lead to a weakening of function or an exhaustion of substance in the long run.

Chinese medicine focuses on treating the person, who happens to be ill; rather than concentrating on the disease mechanism, which happens to be inside a person like is practiced in biomedicine. The treatment methods of Chinese medicine, like other natural medical systems, are not intended to substitute for a bodily function or substance. They are intended to assist the body, help repair any damage, or aid in removing pathogens. When the body is healthy enough to maintain itself, treatment is no longer necessary. As an example, modern research has shown that the common medicinal herbs used to treat infections can not be compared to the potent antibiotics used in hospitals. Many of these herbs can only inhibit the growth of the bacteria, not destroy them. Yet experienced doctors of Chinese medicine will tell you that when properly prescribed, these substances are effective in the treatment of infectious disease, and in chronic cases they are often a better choice than the standard biomedical treatment.

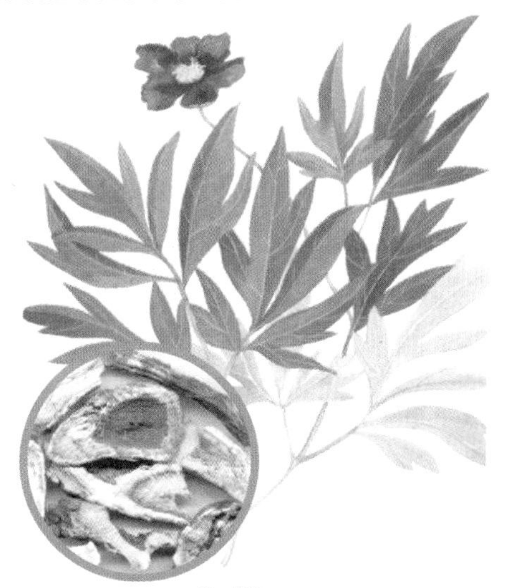

Red Peony

Treatment methods aim to help the body recover by using natural substances and manual methods that stimulate the functions of the body. Eventually, when the body has been "re-trained" to maintain balance on its own, treatment can be reduced and then eliminated. The language it uses, qi, yin-yang, five phases, etc., is antique, but the idea it embraces is timeless.

If you are ready to take an active role in your health and in your life, Chinese medicine is right for you.

But remember, achieving good health is not like climbing a mountain, with a visible goal, but like maintaining a garden, giving constant care and paying attention to changes in the environment. Chinese medicine has been helping transform what is sometimes seen as an arduous task into a rewarding joy for millions of people for thousands of years. If you also want your garden to thrive, come and join the community of natural medicine, learn more about Chinese medicine.

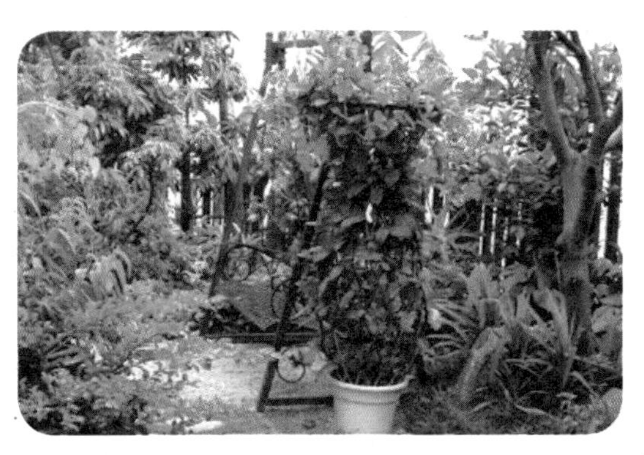

Before introducing detailed information about the theories and treatment methods of Chinese medicine, please read the following legend. It is one that is well known throughout China, revealing the close link Chinese medicine has with the history and folklore of its native land.

Sometime during the Spring and Autumn Period (770 B.C.E. - 476 B.C.E.) or the Warring States Period (476 B.C.E. - 221 B.C.E.), there was a famous doctor named Bian Que. Once, Bian Que traveled to the Kingdom of Gou. When he walked through the palace gates, he overheard that the king's son had just died. He approached someone to ask what the king's son died had from. The doctor was told the young prince had not been able to breathe smoothly for some time, and that recently a sudden stoppage of breath caused his death. Bian Que asked in detail at what time the prince passed away and whether he had yet been placed in a coffin. After getting as many details about the situation as possible, he said solemnly, "Please tell your king, I can bring the prince back to life." The king, upon hearing that someone could rescue his son, was excited and curious. He personally went down to greet Bian Que.

The doctor entered the palace to examine the prince. Once there, he felt the prince's pulse, palpated various parts of his body, and then said to the king enthusiastically, "The prince is not dead but is suffering from a condition called 'body collapse' which resulted from an imbalance of yin and yang. In truth he is not dead; it only seems like death." So the good doctor proceeded to open a small case that contained acupuncture needles, and he needled several points. To the surprise of everyone present, the prince soon stirred and seemed to gain some amount of consciousness. Then Bian Que boiled some herbal medicines, prepared compresses and applied them to the prince's armpits, after which the young man was able to slowly sit up. Within twenty days of taking the medicine the young prince had recovered his health. This news spread far and wide and everyone was saying that Bian Que could bring the dead back to life. From then on Bian Que was called a "supernatural healer".

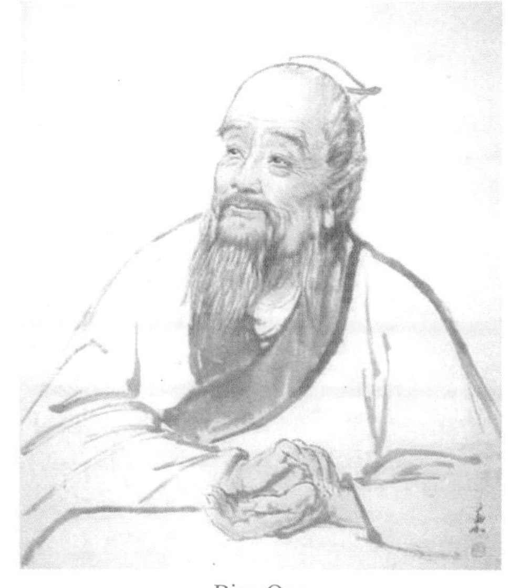

Bian Que

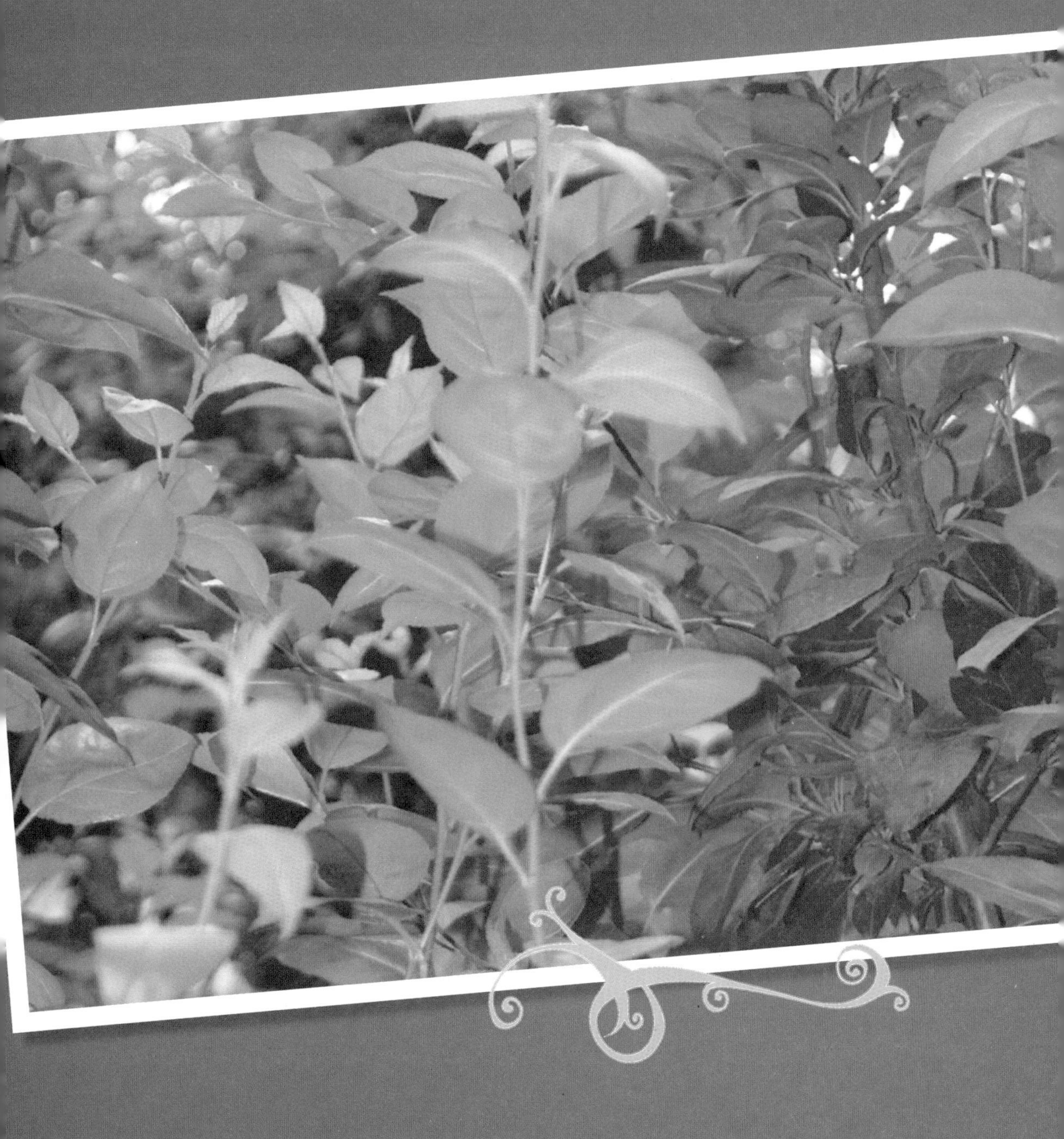

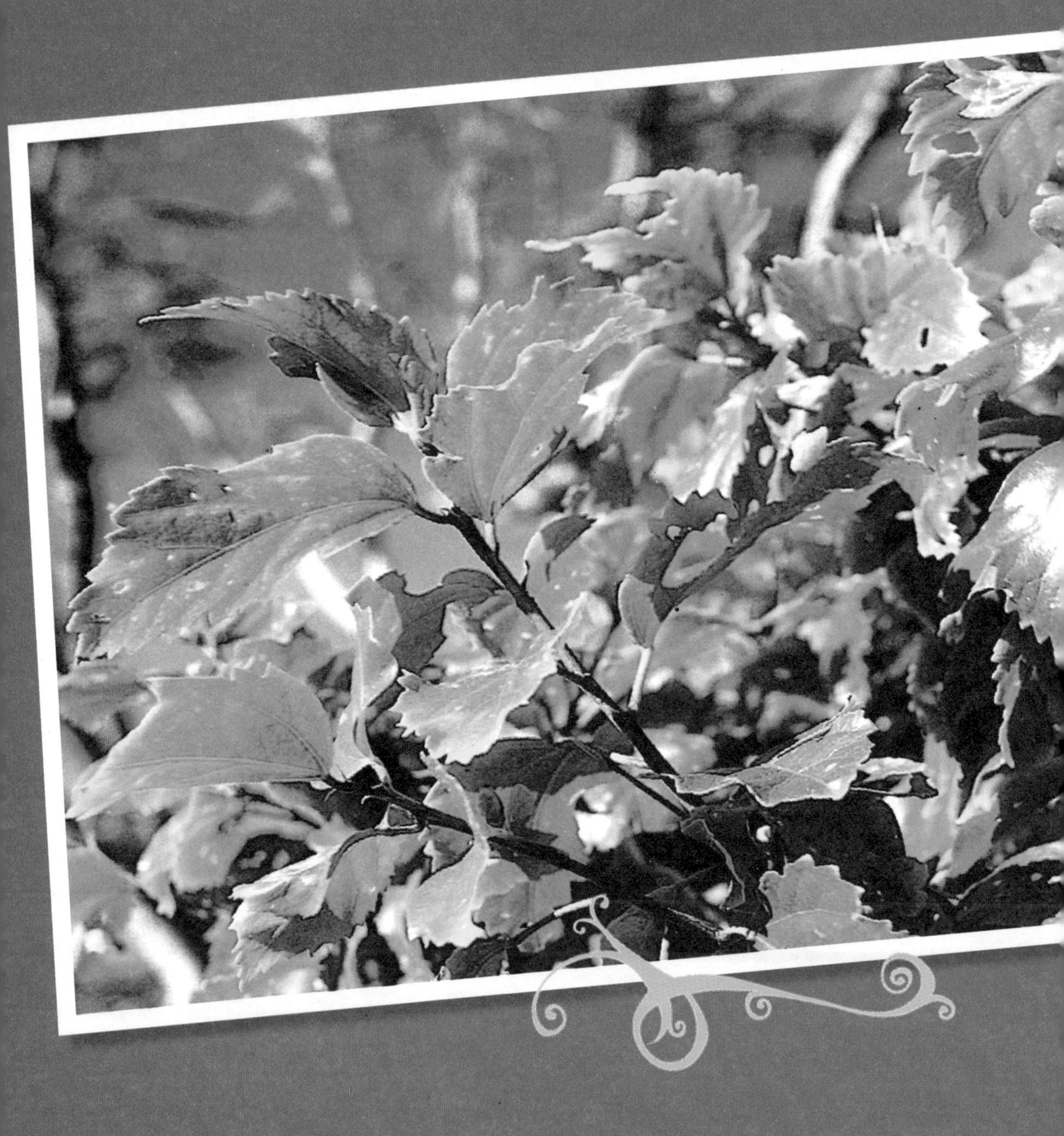

Chapter 2

How Does Chinese Medicine Understand Migraines ?

Some people in Western countries are under the false impression that Chinese medicine and acupuncture involve some kind of sorcery with needles or mysterious spirits. Some religious leaders have even been heard telling their parishioners that it is somehow against their religion or that yin and yang are evil. Though it is true the ancient language of Chinese medi cine can reinforce this view by referring to the "spirits" of the heart, lungs, liver, etc., or by insisting on the existence of the *jīng luò,* which is the channel network that runs throughout the human body and is responsible for transporting qi and blood, to wise doctors and realistic patients, the words used matter little. What is important is if the natural underlying concepts can be used and beneficial results obtained.

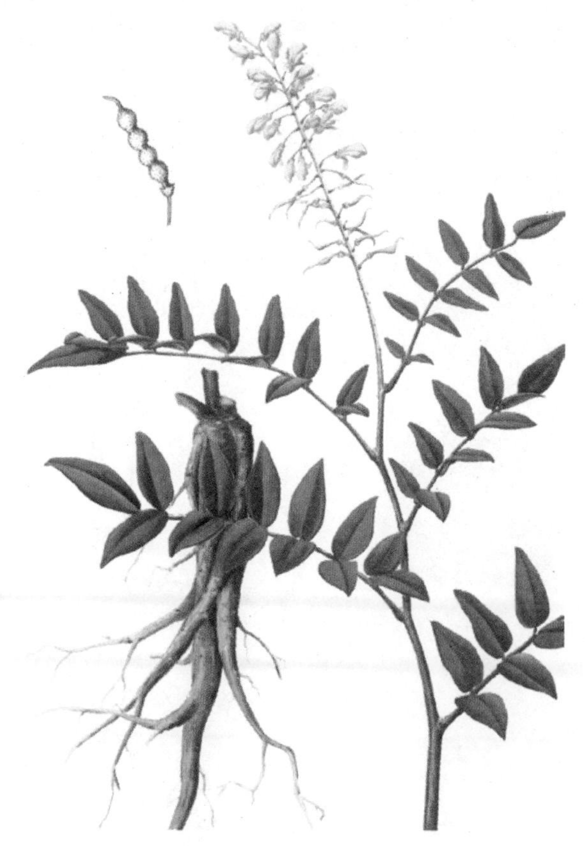

Bushy Sophora

Introduction to Chinese Medicine

Chinese Medicine enjoys a rich tradition and the longest continuous history among the world's natural medicines, with the possible exception of the Indian Ayurvedic tradition. Written legends suggest a history of 5,000 years, while archeological evidence dates back to 1,700 B.C.E. The earliest existing literature dates from 200 B.C.E., but because it includes an organized system of medical material, we know the concepts are from even earlier times. Chinese medicine is remarkable in having not only survived, but thrived during thousands of years of political and social ups-and-downs, and in remaining relevant by continuing to grow, despite the rise of biomedicine. It presently provides safe and effective care at an increasing rate to people all over the world.

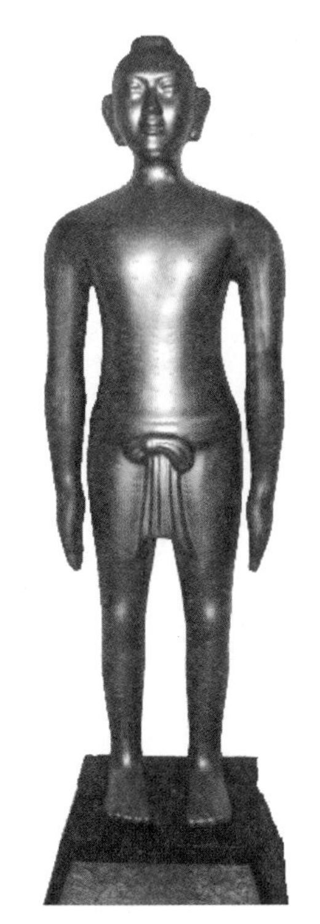

Bronze Acupuncture Model

Perhaps an illustrative example of how Chinese medicine has greatly bene fited society at large will help you understand its potential value to the world. During the infamous influenza epidemic of 1918 that swept over the world causing millions of deaths, the death rate in China was lower than in other countries[11]. It is estimated that over 2% of the world's population died from the flu with some countries suffering as much as a 20% loss of life[12]. The statistics on China's southern province of Guangdong, however, say only 0.1% of the population died[11]. During this time, biomedical treatment was largely unavailable to the vast majority of China's huge population. The people relied on the methods and theories of Chinese medicine to maintain health and treat disease. It is incredible to think that this natural system of health care was effective against one of the deadliest, most rapidly spreading diseases in the past century. Today, Chinese medicine is expected to play a role in providing emergency treatments to combat a similar potential outbreak of avian bird flu.

1. The Beginnings of Chinese Medicine

Like all other world medicines, Chinese medicine developed and expanded mainly through practice and experience. Over 4,000 years ago, the Chinese created medicinal practices during their struggle with nature. They found that particular food or plants could somehow relieve or eliminate a disease. The knowledge of that food or plant was passed down orally until the advent of writing. In utilizing fire for warmth, they found that applying warm stones to certain parts of the body could relieve pain or bring relief From other complaints. In time, they developed methods for using hot compresses and moxibustion. While using stones as tools they found that when a part of the body was mistakenly poked or stabbed, the disorder in another part was relieved. Hence, they created methods of using fine stone or bone "needles" for specific ailments. Through experiences like these, acupuncture was developed, and this further evolved into acupuncture channel theory.

Two thousand years ago the earliest known Chinese medicine book, the *Yellow Emperor's Inner Classic (Huáng Dì Nèi Jīng)*, was written. This book summarizes many medical theories of that time period and then provides instruction on therapeutic treatments. Assimilating achievements of other natural sciences at that time such as seasonal observations, proper nutrition and patterns of aging, it comprehensively examines the physiology and pathology of the body, along with diagnosis, prevention and treatment of diseases. It created a foundation of Chinese medical theory.

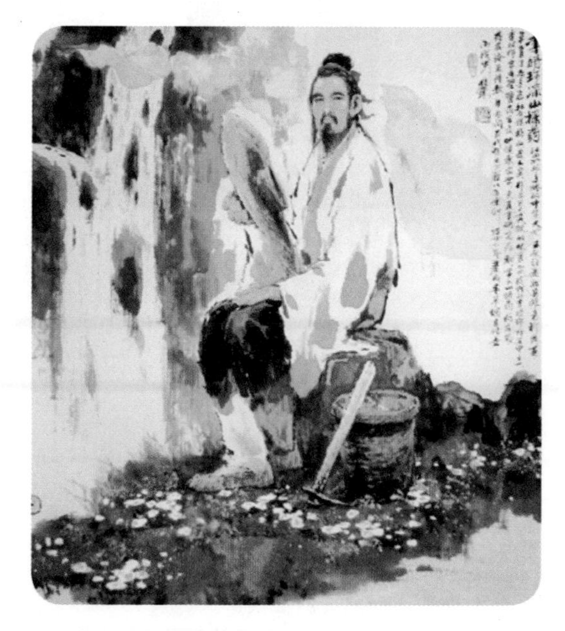

2. The Famous Physician Zhang Zhong-jing

In the development of traditional Chinese medicine, one of the most important persons was a man named Zhang Zhong-jing. He created treatment strategies based on identifiable patterns which developed into the system used by modern Chinese medicine to recognize and treat disease.

Zhang Zhong-jing lived during the Eastern Han Dynasty (25 C.E. – 220 C.E.). He specialized in the study of what he called "cold damage" and other contagious diseases after an epidemic decimated his own family. Doctor Zhang's extended family had more than 200 members. Two thirds of them died from disease within 10 years, 70% of which were from cold damage. The so-called "cold damage" includes what we distinguish today as cholera, dysentery, pneumonia, influenza and some other acute contagious diseases. In the late period of the Eastern Han Dynasty most doctors felt helpless when faced with these diseases. As a result, thousands of people lost their lives.

For that reason, Zhang Zhong-jing labored for several years to develop a complete system of theory that covered pathology, diagnosis, therapy and prescriptions for these problems. He theorized that cold damage developed gradually from an initial attack until the crucial state just before death. Treatment should be varied according to the individual's signs and symptoms at the different stages of disease development. This fundamental principle is the backbone of all treatments and is what is meant by saying Chinese medicine treats the whole person. This individualism whereby two patients with seemingly similar conditions can be treated quite differently from one another contrasts greatly with biomedicine, which tends to treat large swaths of the population identically. Biomedicine thrives on conformity and uniformity while Chinese medicine gains its strength through indi-

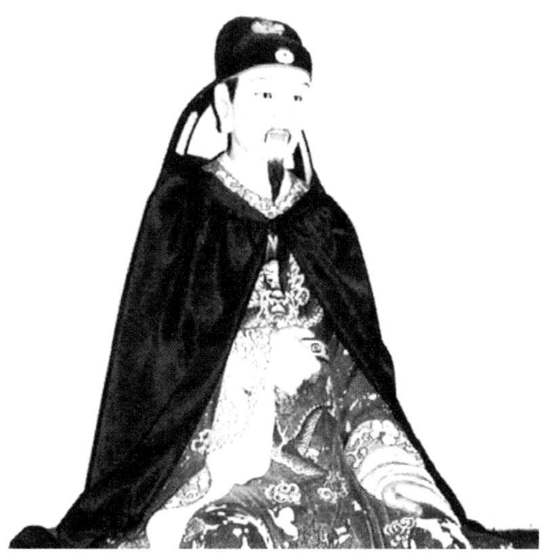

Zhang Zhong-jing

vidualism. This principle also has ensured that Chinese medicine has remained viable from generation to generation. Zhang Zhong-jing detailed his clinical experience while he was practicing medicine, noting down the most effective prescriptions. Based on his years of practical experience, he worked out a monograph, *Annotation to Treatise on Cold-Induced Diseases (Zhù Jiě Shāng Hán Lùn)*. This work is considered a classic of Chinese medicine and Zhang Zhong-jing has been admired as a medical sage for nearly two millennia in honor of his significant contribution to Chinese medicine.

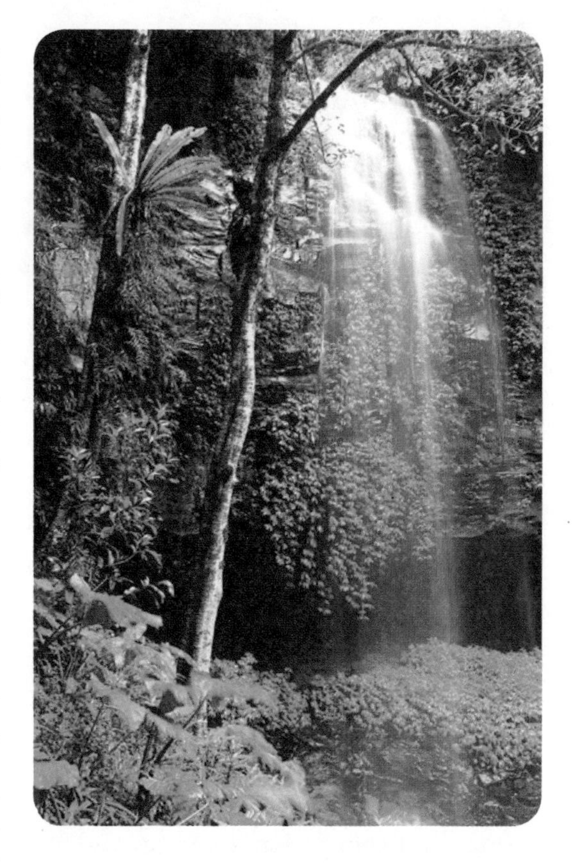

3. The Concept of Holism

Holism means a combination of unity and integrity. No matter the location of the disease, Chinese medicine pays attention to the entire body as well as to the relationship between the human body and the external environment. The human body itself is seen as an organic whole, every part cooperates and influences the rest. The idea of unity between interior and exterior conditions and the entirety of the body itself is essential to the concept of holism. Humans are tied to nature, and in nature there exists the essential conditions for human life. Changes in nature, therefore, may directly or indirectly influence the body, and accordingly cause reactions that may result in disease.

4. Treatment Based on Patterns

Treatment based on patterns is an essential principle and characteristic of Chinese medicine's understanding and treatment of disease. It should be noted that a "pattern" is a summary of the cause, location and nature of a disease, and an evaluation of the conflict between the external

pathogenic factors and the body's resistance. Pattern differentiation includes analyzing signs and symptoms into various patterns of disharmony. Treatment is then decided based on the patterns identified. Pattern differentiation is the prerequisite and basis for determining that treatment. If treatment is effective, this confirms for the doctor that the patterns identified were correct.

Treatment based on patterns differs from symptomatic treatment and treatment according to disease, which are the primary methods of biomedicine. While both are valid methods of determining treatment, the style of pattern identification used in Chinese medicine allows for a more flexible approach to diagnosis and treatment. As an example, a person may suffer from headaches for years, but due to changes in the person's diet, lifestyle, and living environment, the patterns present and therefore the treatments administered will also vary. This is why patients with the same disease but different patterns should be treated differently. A traditional Chinese practitioner sees layers of patterns within the same disease.

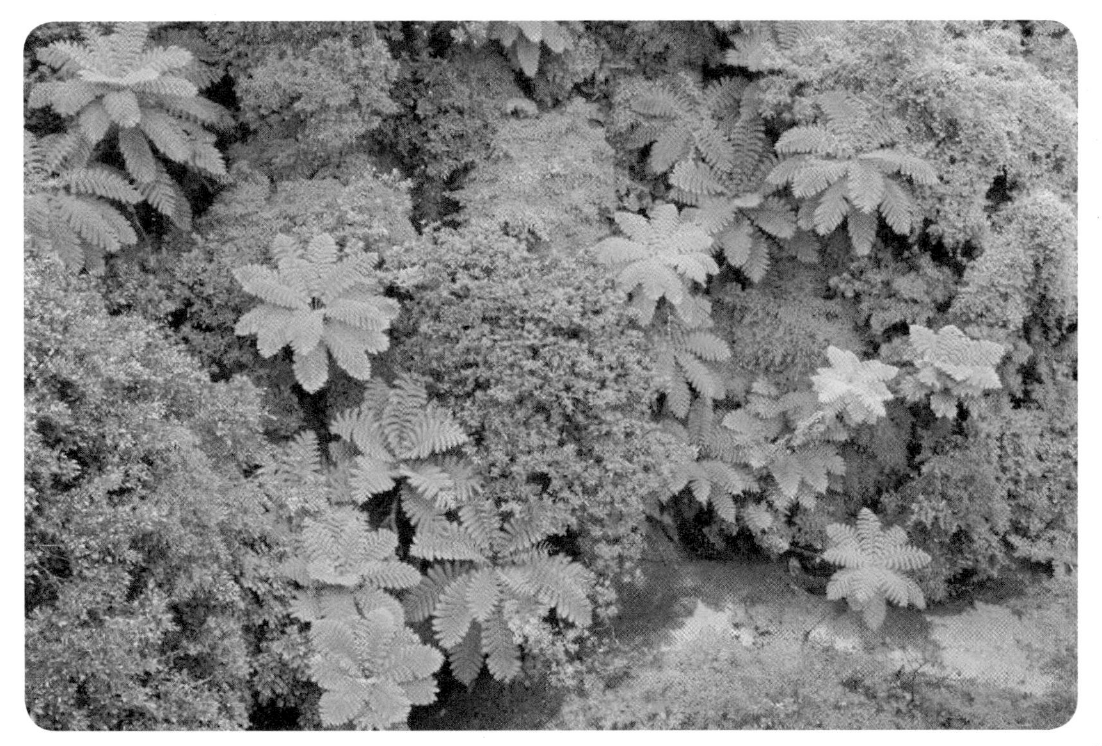

Three Key Concepts in Chinese Medicine

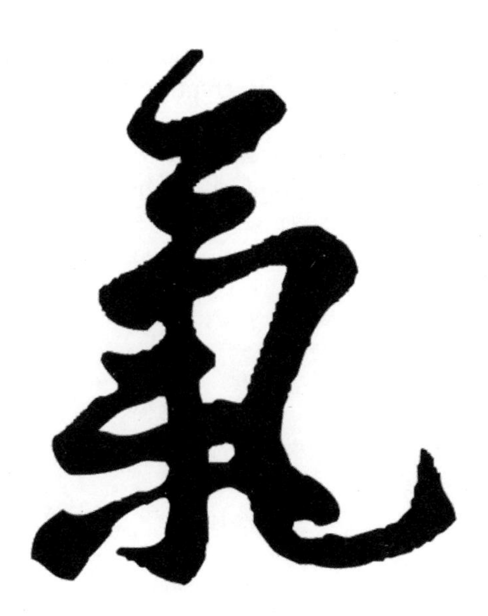

1. Qi

The concept of qi is much more than a medical term. Indeed, it is inseparable from ancient Chinese philosophy and is used by both fields to explain the forces that animate and control everything in the universe, from the cycle of seasons, to the origins and effects of emotions, to the inner workings of the human body. There is no simple literal English translation of qi. Different translators have rendered it as air, vapor, or energy and all of these are partially, but not completely, accurate.

The concept of qi is somewhat similar to *pneuma* in ancient Greece or *prana* in India, which were used to describe an underlying life force that was seen as having a strong connection to air and breath. Some of qi's important characteristics are:

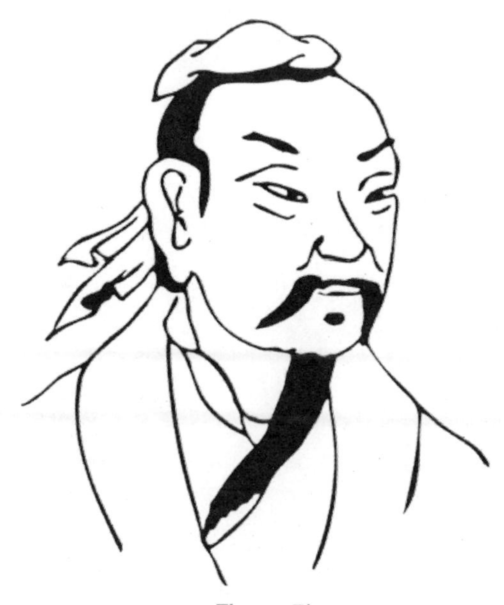

Zhuang Zi

- Qi is a kind of life force, but it is also a tangible vital substance that makes up everything in the cosmos, including humans.

- Qi is the medium for transformation that stimulates the process of change. Everything in the universe, organic or inorganic, is made of qi and defined by qi. Mountains, rivers, animals, plants, even human emotions all have qi.

- Qi cannot be defined as simply "energy", nor can it be labeled a mere material substance, nor is it something in between. It is what connects humankind and the natural environment.

- Qi is the media that makes the relationships and interactions between things and lives possible.

It can be difficult to understand the ancient Chinese claim that qi is both an ethereal life force as well as a material substance. To understand better, let us look at two very different categories of phenomena: human emotions and simple writing utensils, and see how qi exists in both of them.

First, take emotions. If a doctor of Chinese medicine was asked to describe the qi of the emotion joy, he or she would probably say that its qi was light, rising, dispersing or possibly warm. On the other hand, if asked to describe the qi of fear, the words used would be more along the lines of dark, sinking, or cold. These descriptions are not based on any lab tests or scientific evidence, but are based primarily on the practitioner's own experience of the resonance between the emotional state and his or her perception.

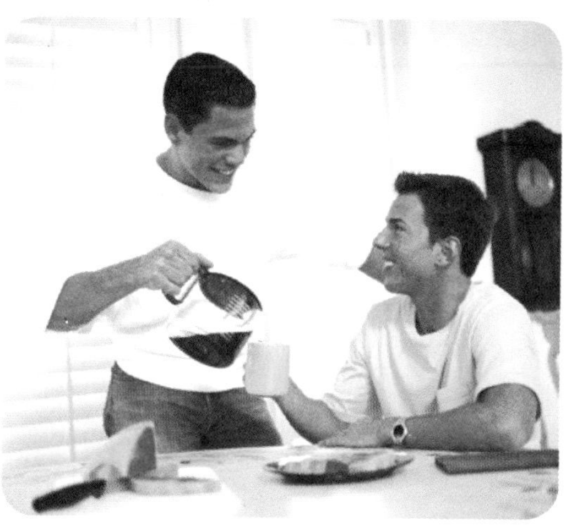

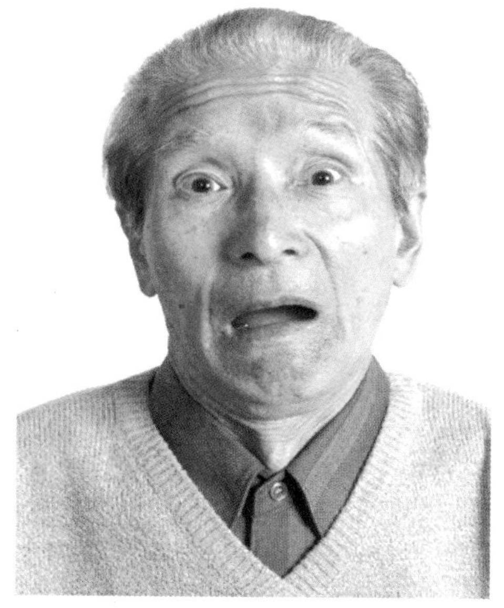

Now let us look at the other end of the spectrum using two examples of solid, tangible writing utensils. One, a well-worn wooden pencil bearing teeth-marks and a cartoon character design, the kind of pencil a first-grader might use to scratch out the ABC's; the other, a sleek, expensive ink pen, probably black or silver that could be used to sign legal contracts. Similar to the description of joy above, the qi of the pencil could be described as light, familiar, or warm; and similar to the qi of fear above, the pen's qi would be described as dark, heavy, and cold.

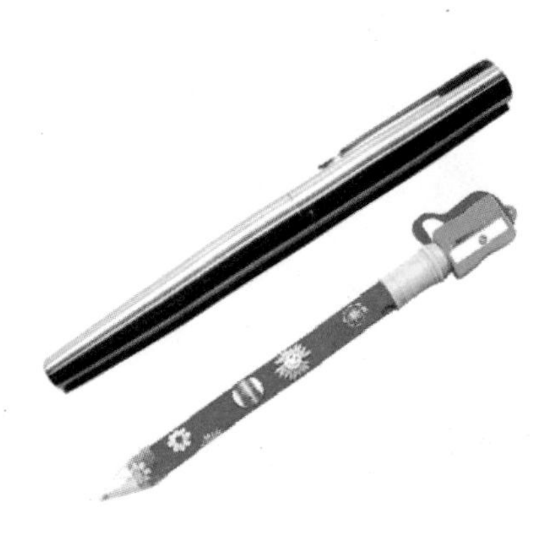

We can see that qi is not merely energy, as the physical substances of the pen and pencil were crucial parts to describing their qi. Likewise, we saw that qi cannot be limited to physical characteristics because the emotions described above, which have their distinct qi, have no tangible substance.

Chinese medicine, over thousands of years and with the help of countless doctors, patients, and philosophers has established a system in which the different phenomena of the universe can be described by qi and likewise the relationships between these phenomena can be described. Thus a practitioner, when asked to describe the qi of something or the other, is not merely relying on his own experience and perceptions, but is using established theories to come up with an accurate description that anyone trained in qi will be able to agree with. In fact, it does not necessarily take training to understand qi. Most people would find the metaphorical descriptions of joy, fear, the pencil, and the pen easy to relate to. All people can think and talk in terms of qi, since it is based on the common sense of the natural world. The genius of Chinese medicine lies in its clear definitions and natural categorizations.

To understand what doctors of Chinese medicine aim to do in their treatments, we have to understand this well-used but rarely understood word, qi. In Chinese medicine, qi is subdivided into dozens of different functions with correlating descriptions, such as "defensive qi", "digestive qi" and terms which might require greater explanation such as *yíng qì* or *zhèng q*. Matter and energy are not independent of each other, as there is an intrinsic relationship between them. Qi is a concept of both matter and energy. It is the force that animates life. It is also the

matter that constitutes life. Qi is shared by everything in the universe. It is the medium by which interactions take place. To quote one of the original textbooks of Chinese medicine in English, *The Web That Has No Weaver* by Ted Kapchuk:

"The interaction, or resonance, is realized by qi. Health is the harmonious resonance while disease is the disharmony. Components of the universe, the qi of herbs (plants, animal parts, and stones), acupuncture points (junctions of the human network), lifestyle activities (movement, rest, food and relationships) or living environments (seasons, weather, or even air conditioning) share a resonating frequency that already exists in a person. A medicine or a conscious shift in a person's behavior can resonate with the condition within a person (e.g. a pattern of a disharmony) and induce a person toward health."

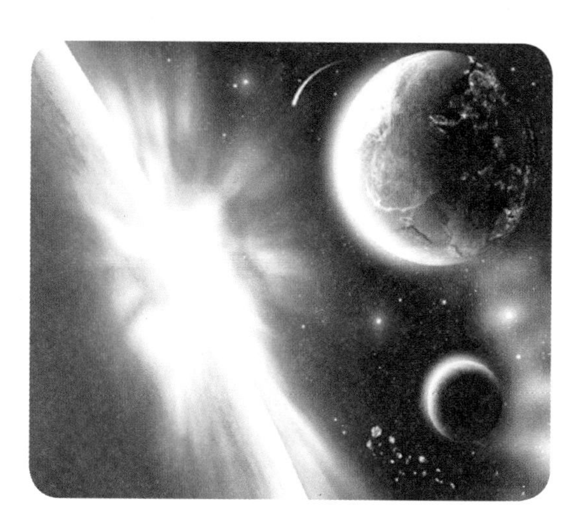

Functions of qi

In terms of the human body and its various activities, Chinese medicine describes qi as having five major attributes. They are as follows.

★ Promoting

Just as wind, which is simply highly active air, provides energy to push the sails of a boat or turn the turbine of a windmill, qi provides the active, vital energy necessary for the growth and development of the human body and to perform the functions of the organs, channels and tissues. In addition, qi promotes the formation and circulation of blood and supports the metabolism of body fluids. If there is a deficiency of qi, its promoting functions are weakened. As a result, growth and development can be affected or delayed, the organs and channels cannot function properly and blood formation is hampered, leading to a series of health problems.

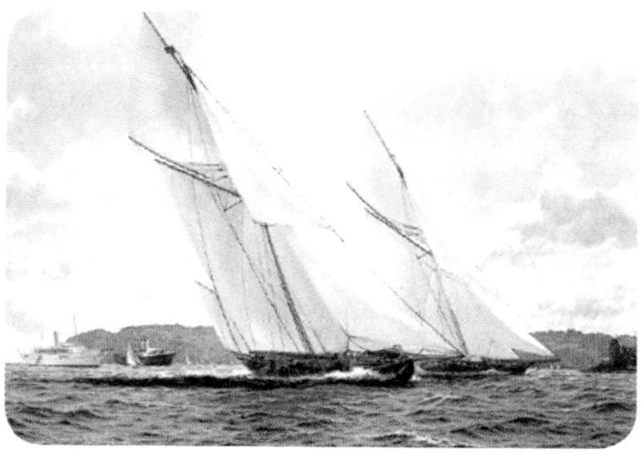

★ Warming

In a gaseous state, air contains more kinetic heat energy than in its liquid state. Like air, qi also contains heat energy for the body. Being a heat source, qi warms the body and keeps it at a constant temperature so normal bodily functions can take place. Deficiency of qi can lead to a lowered body temperature, intolerance of cold and cold hands and feet.

★ Defending

In Chinese medicine, one of the main causes of disease is invasion by what are called "external evils". These "evils" are simply environmental factors that can lead to illness. The six traditional evils are wind, summer heat, dampness, dryness, cold and fire. One particular type of qi resists the entry of these external evils, defending the body and maintaining health. In scientific terms, this defense qi acts like the immune system.

★ Consolidation and retention

Qi helps to retain the various bodily substances and also keeps the organs in their proper place. Qi keeps the blood flowing within the vessels and prevents it from leaking out into the tissues. It controls the secretion and excretion of sweat, urine and saliva, and keeps body fluids from escaping the body. Qi also consolidates and stores sperm to prevent premature ejaculation. Finally, qi consolidates the organs and stops them from descending into a position where they cannot function properly. If qi is deficient, the consolidating function is weakened, leading to various health problems such as bleeding problems, frequent urination, premature ejaculation and uterine or kidney prolapse (where the organ sinks).

The promoting and consolidating functions work in a complementary manner. For example, qi promotes blood circulation and the distribution of body fluids, but it also controls and adjusts these same substances. The balance between these two functions is essential for maintaining healthy blood circulation and water metabolism.

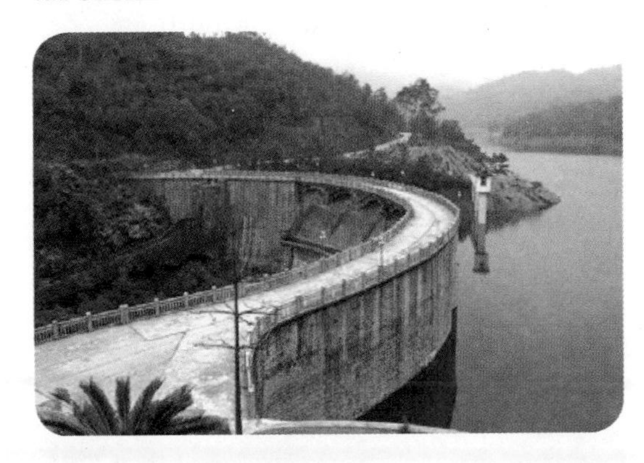

★ Transforming

The functions of transformation are important for the metabolism of fundamental substances. As suggested by these words, qi may "vaporize" substances in the body and transform them into essence or vital energy. For example, certain actions of qi allow food to be changed into food essence, which is in turn transformed into different types of qi and blood. Indigestible food and waste are also transformed by qi into urine and stool to be excreted.

Movements of qi

The four directions of qi movement are: up, down, out and in. These movements are so important that once qi can no longer travel in these directions, life will come to an end.

Each organ has different specialized movements. It is important to note that many terms in Chinese medicine cannot be literally translated into English. Qi was a previous example, and now we reach the word "spleen". To Chinese medicine, the single word spleen is meant to denote a much more varied function than what is identified as spleen in biomedical anatomy. For example, spleen qi ascends the pure part of digested food from the stomach for transformation into nutritional essence. Stomach qi, on the other hand, pushes food downward to the intestines in order to remove its impurities. Some organs, like the lungs, perform movements in all four directions. Lung qi moves in and out during breathing. However, when disseminating nutritional essence to the body, lung qi may ascend to reach the upper portions of the body and then descend where it is said the kidneys "grasp the lung qi" for further energy.

The different movements of qi work in a coordinated manner to maintain a harmonious balance. The ascending balances the descending movement while the outward balances the inward movement. Balanced movement is important for promoting the functions of different tissues, organs and channels. Disharmonious movement of qi leads to health problems. For example, insufficient downward movement of lung qi causes a cough. When stomach qi cannot properly descend, nausea and vomiting occurs. This type of condition is called "rebellious qi."

Types of qi

Qi is further classified according to its type. The four main types are inborn qi, pectoral qi, nutritive qi and protective qi.

★ Inborn qi

Inborn qi is the original, essential and vital qi that possesses prenatal and congenital properties. After conception, "congenital essence" (essential vital substances inherited from parents, essentially hereditary factors) is stored by the kidneys, the place from which inborn qi originates. Inborn qi is further nourished by "acquired essence" of the spleen and stomach. These are essences and energies derived mainly from food and drink, but also from respiration and rest. After this process is complete, inborn qi is ready to travel through the entire body to exert its effects. Starting from the portion between the two kidneys, known as the "vital gate", the qi circulates through the organs, muscles, skin and channels providing the power for all of life's activities.

★ Pectoral qi

Pectoral qi is stored in the chest. It is formed by combining fresh air inhaled by the lungs and food essence derived from the spleen and the stomach. Because pectoral qi concentrates in the chest, it can penetrate the blood vessels of the heart and lungs and move outward during expiration and inward during inspiration. By flowing through the respiratory tract, pectoral qi supports the breathing function of the lungs and affects the strength of the voice. Its ability to flow through the blood vessels and the heart is important in regulating the heartbeat and supporting the circulation of other types of qi and blood. Pectoral qi also plays a role in keeping the body warm and influences the activities of the limbs.

★ Nutritive qi

Nutritive qi, as its name suggests, supplies nourishment to the body. It mainly circulates through the blood vessels with the blood. Sometimes this combination of nutritive qi and blood is referred to collectively as "nutritive blood". Nutritive qi mainly comes from food essence derived by the spleen and stomach's transformation and transportation properties. Starting from these organs, nutritive qi goes to the lungs where it enters the circulation. Nutritive qi has yin properties so it can form into materials needed by other parts of the body. For example, its close relationship with blood allows it to provide some of the necessary substances needed to produce new blood. Nutritive qi also provides necessary nutrients to support the functions of the organs.

★ Protective qi

Protective qi protects against external evils or pathogens. As previously mentioned, evils are environmental factors that lead to illness. Unlike nutritive qi, protective qi has yang properties, because it has more functional characteristics.

Protective qi also comes from food essence derived by the spleen and stomach. It moves outside the blood vessels and circulates in different areas than nutritive qi. Internally, protective qi is distributed to the diaphragm and scattered around the chest and abdominal cavities. Externally, it moves between the skin and muscles providing protection. Protective qi not only guards against illness and disease but also regulates the sweat glands and pores and provides nourishment for skin, hair and muscles.

Although nutritive and protective qi share the same origin, their flow directions, as previously described, are opposite to one another. By balancing their nutritive (yin) and protective (yang) functions, healthy sweating, temperature control and defense functions are maintained.

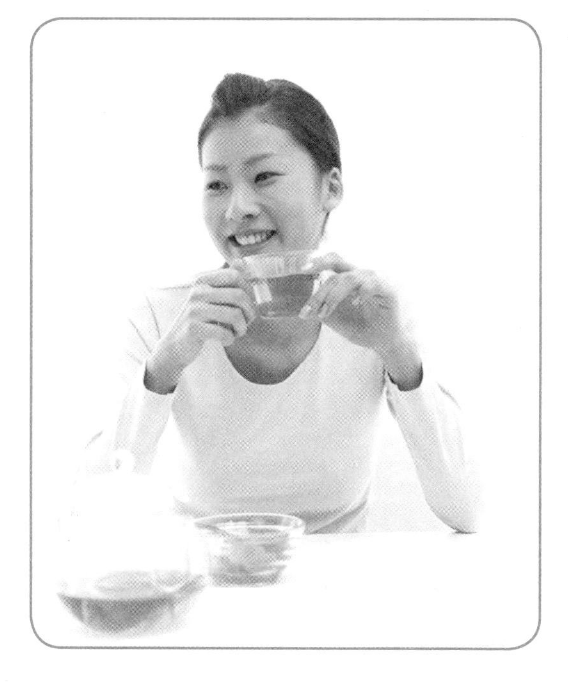

The relationship between qi and blood

According to traditional Chinese medical theory, qi is the supreme commander of blood, and blood is the mother of qi. Blood will not flow without qi while qi maintains its form with the help of the blood. These two substances are closely related. Generally there are four primary components to the qi / blood relationship.

★ Qi generates blood.

According to Chinese medicial theory, blood is made from essential qi extracted from food by the spleen and stomach. Thus, when qi is deficient, sufficient blood will not be produced.

★ Qi moves the blood.

The lung qi along with heart qi command the qi and blood respectively and together are responsible for propeling the blood through the vessels.

★ Qi holds the blood.

The spleen qi is responsible for the structural integrity of the body, including the capacity of the vessels to hold the blood and keep it from leaking out.

★ Blood nourishes qi.

Blood serves to anchor the qi and helps prevent qi from rising upward. Blood also provides nutrition and sustains the qi, thus it is said, "Blood is the mother of qi." Again, it is worth mentioning that qi can transform into blood and blood can transform into qi.

In summary, qi is the power behind the supply of blood in the circulatory system. Qi is the driving force of the heart and makes the blood flow. Qi is the general force that animates the body's functions. Qi and blood are also the material basis on which different parts of the body can interact. When our qi and blood are healthy and plentiful, we enjoy physical and emotional well-being. This healthy qi and blood can be easily disrupted if health is neglected. These disruptions can be caused by sudden weather changes, stress, unhealthy food, unhappy relationships, or lack of proper physical activity.

The function of blood and qi is extremely important for the head, brain and central nervous system, which is called the *Sea of Marrow* in Chinese medicine. With enough well circulating qi and blood the nervous system gets enough nutrition to facilitate normal mental functions. Chinese medicine understands the nervous system controls normal functions of every tissue and organ in the body, and without the brain's accurate and sensitive command, our life would be in chaos.

The basis of physiology, pathology, diagnosis, and treatment in Chinese medicine is the theory of essential qi and blood. This theory's main principle is that essential qi and blood are the fundamental substances which constitute the body. Physiological and pathological changes in the body result from normal and abnormal movements of qi and blood respectively. Analyzing the movements of qi and blood is an essential part of diagnosis in Chinese medicine, which is called pattern differentiation. Therefore, the purpose of treatment is to recognize and then adjust abnormalities of qi and blood.

For example, some migraine headache patients complain of feelings of fullness in their head, a bitter taste in the mouth, irritability and ringing in the ears. Biomedicine can not offer reasonable explanations why these symptoms are found together. But Chinese medicine can. The collection of these symptoms falls under the category of excessive ris-

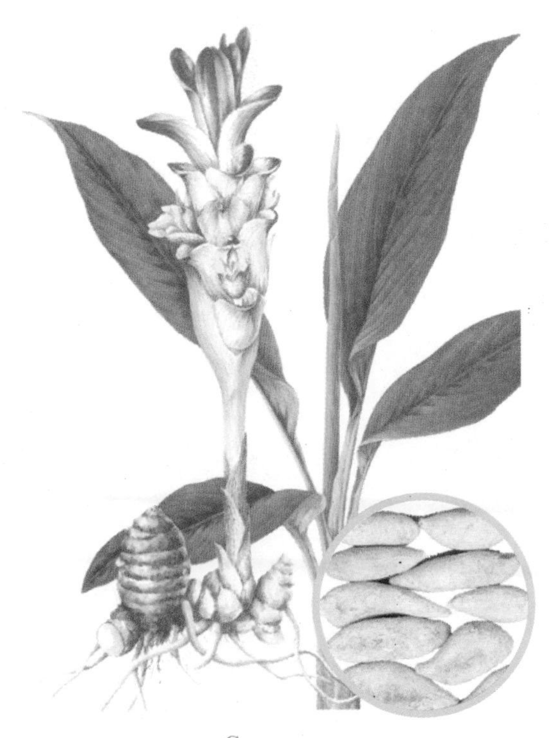

Curcuma

ing of liver yang. Fullness of the head is caused when liver qi rises into the head uncontrollably. Likewise, bitter taste in the mouth, irritability and tinnitus may all be caused by abnormal movement of liver yang. Picture an image of a hot pot on the stove with too much fire beneath it. That excess fire is burning the contents of the pot and releasing steam or vapor violently upwards. Depending on what is cooking, it may smell bad – thus the bitter taste in the mouth. When this kind of migraine patient receives treatment, they may be given medicinal substances which pacify the liver and disperse the liver qi, such as curcuma or bupleurum.

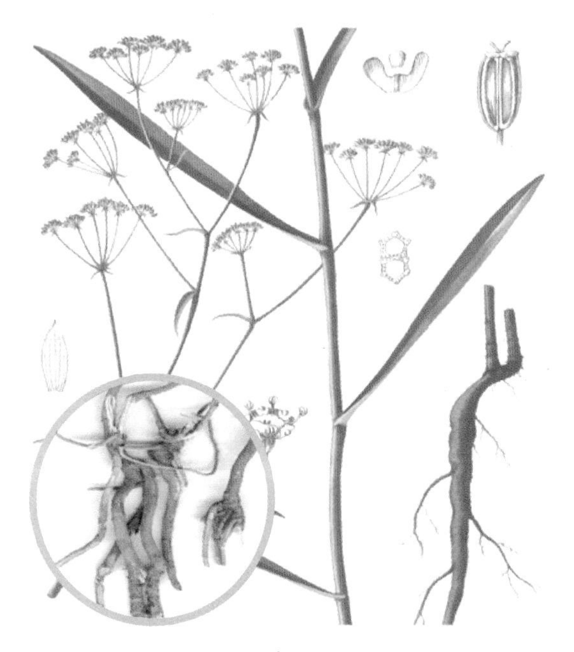

Bupleurum

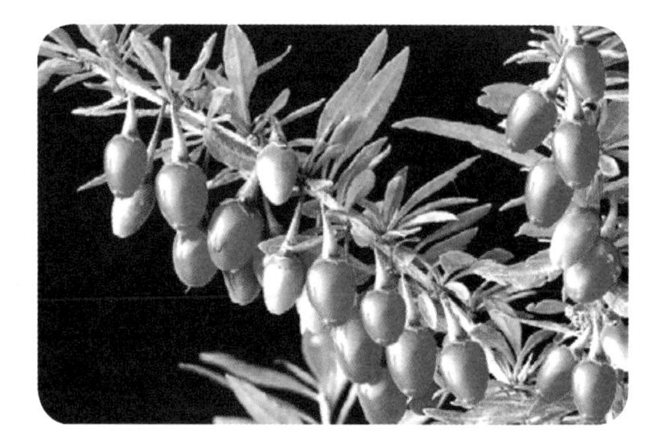

The meaning of qi is many faceted. Qi is what links humans to nature; it is the material basis for all things. Chinese medicine has discovered through centuries of close clinical observation that the qi of the internal organs can be reflected on external parts of the body. By observing external manifestations, the functions of the internal organs can be inferred. Meanwhile, stimulus received externally can be conducted into the internal organs by qi. Acupuncture, moxibustion and massage are all based on the concept that qi in the channels can act on the internal organs.

The fundamental, simple concepts are most important and often neglected in learning. The idea of qi, along with yin-yang theory, is of utmost importance to Chinese medicine. Without qi there is death; with qi there is life. Try not to form a fixed idea about these concepts after only this short explanation. Keep an open mind and deepen your understanding of qi as we explore more about Chinese medicine.

Case 1

Ms. Lin was a 35 year old patient who had suffered from migraine headaches for several years. At the age of 33, blood vessel occlusions in the head were confirmed by MRI examination. Upon learning this she became disappointed with her current treatments and stopped them. She had taken all kinds of pain-killing medications, but without lasting results, and intense side-effects troubled her daily life. The paroxysmal frequency of the migraines increased during the previous year, so she finally decided to try Chinese medicine for relief. Dr. Qin diagnosed her with stagnation of qi due to depression of the liver; the extreme pain was due to blood stasis. Normal movement of qi in Lin's body had been troubled due to a long-term illness which started a cycle of metabolic problems. Because the liver qi was not smooth, the circulation of blood was also not smooth, and this in turn caused blood stasis in the channels that travel through the head. Professor Qin's prescription used a large dosage of medicinals for relieving qi stagnation in the liver and regulating the overall flow of blood. Ms. Lin was also put back on a small dosage of a pain-killer by her doctor. After taking the formula for several months her symptoms improved, and migraines did not occur frequently. Her sleep quality also improved. Very pleased with the result, Ms. Lin will continue taking a small dose of the herbal formula to consolidate the effect of treatment over time.

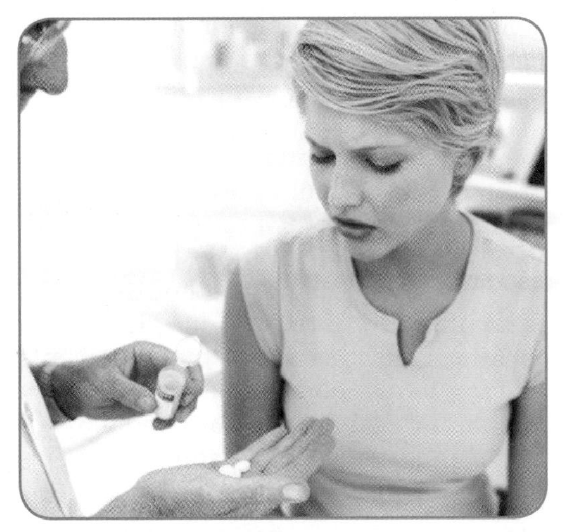

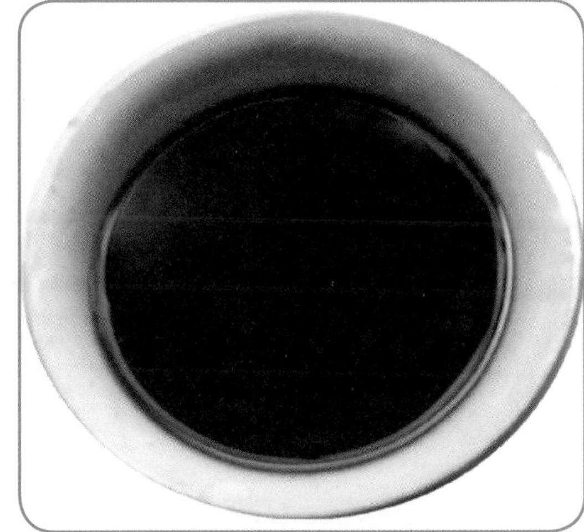

2. Yin – Yang

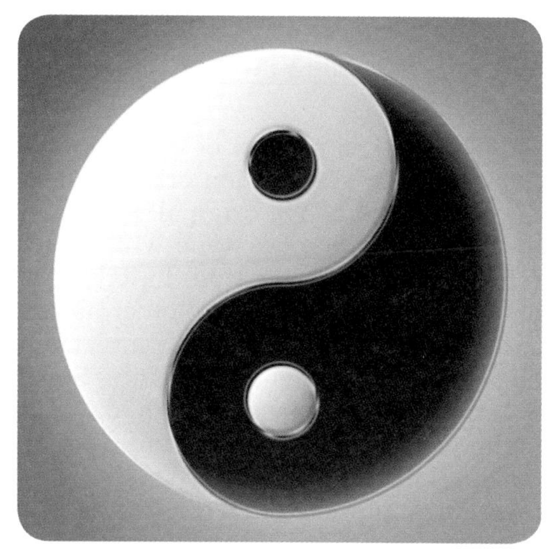

Ancient Chinese people were greatly interested in the relationships and patterns that occurred in nature. Instead of studying isolated subjects, they viewed the world as a harmonious and holistic entity. In their eyes, no single being or object could exist unless it was seen in relation to its surrounding environment. By simplifying these relationships, they tried to explain complicated phenomena of the universe.

Yin-yang theory is a kind of logic which views things in relation to their whole. The theory is based on two basic components: yin and yang (pronounced *yáng*), which combine in a complementary manner and form a method for explaining relationships between objects. Gradually, this logic was developed into a system of thought that was applied to all areas of early Chinese science and philosophy. Medicine used yin-yang theory to understand complicated relationships in the body.

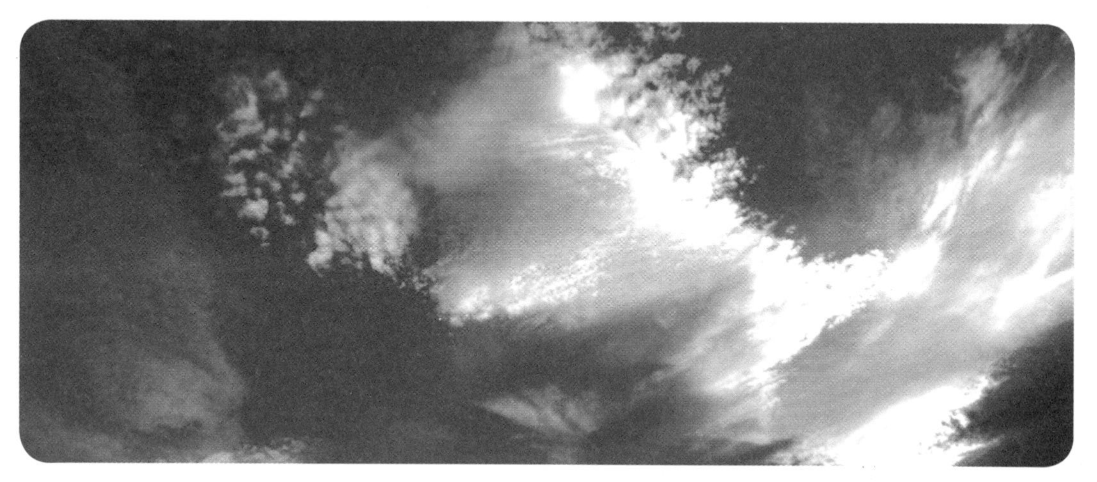

The Origin of the Yin-Yang Theory

The original concept of yin and yang came from the observation of nature and the environment. Yin originally referred to the shady side of a slope while yang referred to the sunny side. Later, these descriptions were applied to other objects and occurrences, to describe complementary and opposing characteristics. Some examples include: sky and earth, day and night, water and fire, active and passive, male and female, and so on. Working with these ideas, our ancestors recognized that all things have yin and yang properties. Yin and yang can describe two relative aspects of the same phenomena such as the example of the different slopes of a mountain, or they can describe two different objects like sky and earth.

Usually, yang is associated with energetic qualities. For example, movement, outward and upward directions, heat, brightness, stimulation, activity and excitement are all yang qualities. Yin, on the other hand, is associated with the physical form of an object and has less energetic qualities such as rest, inward and downward direction, cold, darkness, condensation, inhibition, and nourishment. See the table for a description of yin and yang characteristics.

Categorization of Yin and Yang

Category	Yang	Yin
Time	Day	Night
Space	Heaven	Earth
Season	Spring, Summer	Autumn, Winter
Temperature	Hot	Cold
Weight	Light	Heavy
Speed	Fast	Slow
Motion	Up and out, Vigorous	Down and in, Subtle
Brightness	Light	Dark
Sex	Male	Female
Tissue and organs	Skin, Hair	Bone, Tendon
Disease	Acute	Chronic

In Chinese medicine the fundamental definition of health is when there is a good balance of yin and yang in the body. Diagnosis of disease and its treatment are all aimed at restoring this equilibrium. This may sound simplistic, but when you consider the fact that all organs, functions, emotions, fluids, and structures each have yin and yang aspects that must be balanced, you can see how the doctor's job of detecting every imbalance by using no more than the five senses is a very difficult task.

Yin and yang are interdependent. This means that the condition of one will affect the other. If there is too little yin, then yang will appear to be in excess; and if there is too much yin, there will appear to be too little yang. The reverse is of course true when there is too little or too much yang. A simple example can be seen when the body's temperature rises or falls too much. With a fever there is an overabundance of yang heat. This means the cool yin aspect of the body is not sufficient to counteract the heat. Therefore the prac-

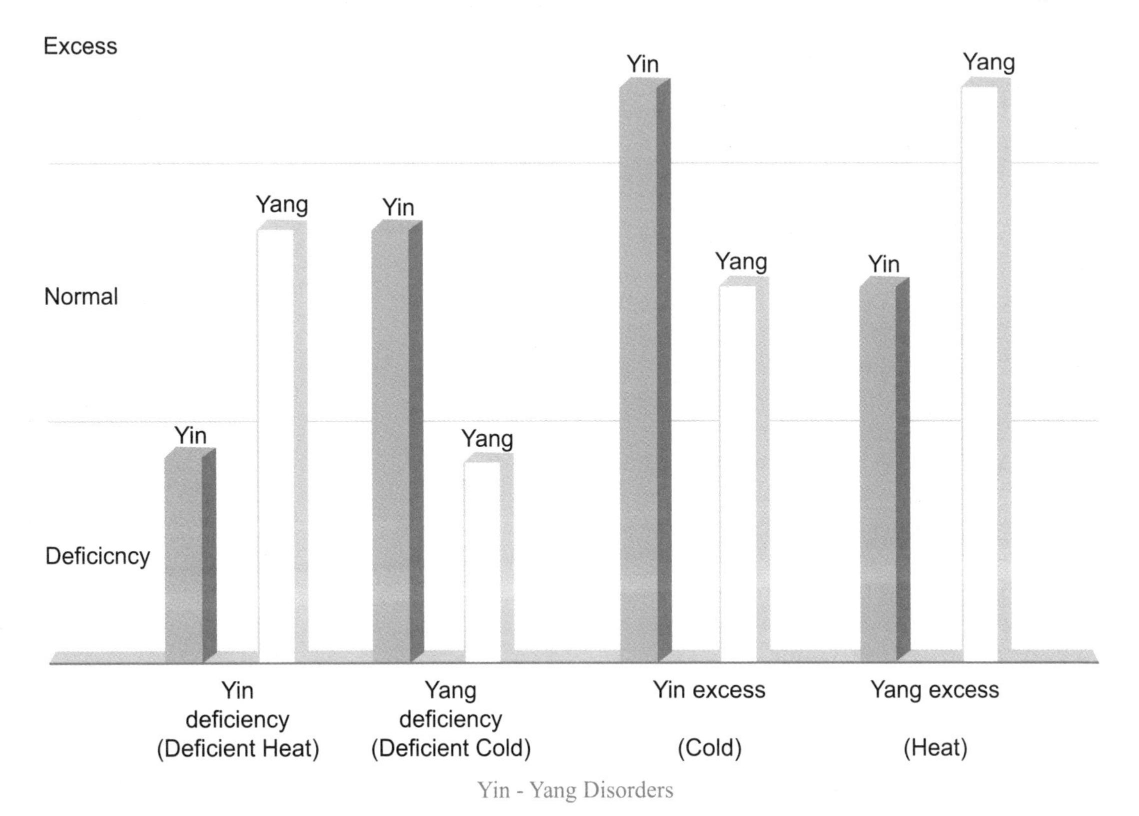

Yin - Yang Disorders

titioner must restore the balance of yin and yang by making the cool yin aspect of the body equal to the hot yang aspect. Likewise, if a patient has hypothermia and has dangerously low body temperature there is a relative abundance of yin cold in relation to yang heat.

However, it is not enough to know merely which is the stronger of yin or yang and which is the weaker. If there is more yang than yin, for example, this could be due to an actual excess of yang and thus yin would be relatively weak, or it could be because there is not enough yin and therefore yang only appears to be in excess. In Chinese medicine these would be called true heat and deficient heat respectively.

This is a difficult concept for all beginning students of Chinese medicine so let us look at an example. A forest that has not had any rain for many months will be dry and probably hot. Dryness and heat are yang qualities as opposed to yin moisture and cold. A forest that is on fire is also in a condition of extreme yang heat. In each case, the yang aspect is greater than the yin aspect. But to restore the yin and yang balance of both situations, one must choose different strategies. To restore the forest in drought it is necessary to add yin, meaning water. On the other hand, to balance a blazing fire, one has no other option but to remove the excess yang fire. In Chinese medicine, the dry forest would be said to be in a state of yin deficiency, where the heat is due to a relative abundance of yang. The forest fire is a state of yang excess, where yin may very well be normal. The other states are yang deficiency and yin excess. Please see the diagrams to better understand the four different types of yin-yang imbalances in the body.

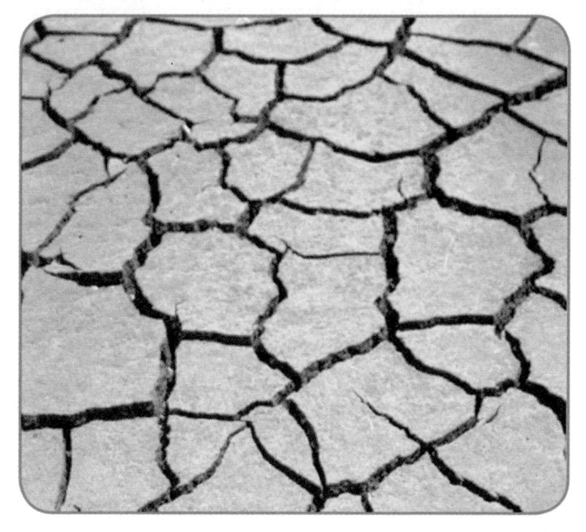

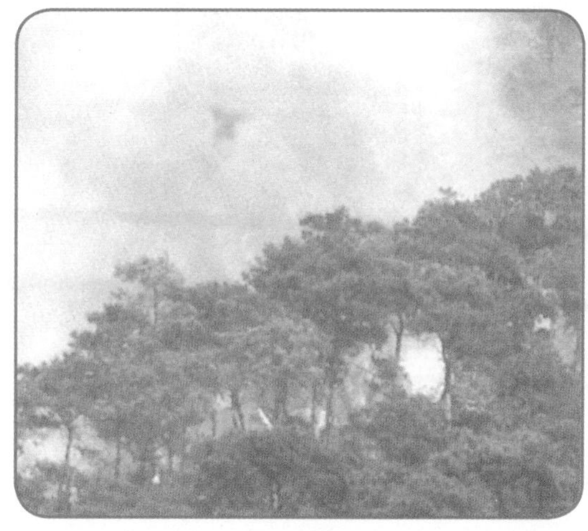

Different Types of Yin - Yang Imbalances

	Typical Manifestations
Yang excess	Fever, aversion to heat, thirst, desire for cold drinks, reddish complexion, restlessnes, yellowish-colored mucus, dark-colored urination, constipation, red tongue, yellowish tongue coating, rapid pulse
Yin excess	Aversion to cold, no thirst, desire for warm drinks, thin and watery mucus, loose stool, pale complexion, light-colored tongue, whitish tongue coating, slow or tense pulse
Yang deficiency	Preference for warmth, cold limbs, pale complexion, spontaneous sweating, fatigue, shortness of breath, loose stool, enlarged and light-colored tongue, whitish tongue coating, deep, slow and weak pulse
Yin deficiency	Thirst, dry mouth and throat, hot feeling in the soles and palms, afternoon fever, night sweating, red tongue with little coating, rapid and fine pulse

With chronic diseases, diagnosis and treatment in Chinese medicine is generally more dynamic than in biomedicine. Conditions may change daily, though with chronic disease it is usually safe to reevaluate once a week or more.

For migraine patients, the typical cause of the disease in Chinese medicine is excessive liver yang that rises and irritates the upper orifices of the head. Typical symptoms include severe head pain that often involves the temples or eye sockets, overall fullness of the head, moodiness with emotional outbursts, insomnia and bitterness in the mouth. Additional signs and symptoms may result if the headaches are chronic, frequent or if there are drug side-effects. And if one considers the fact that most pharmaceutial drugs for migraines injure the liver over time, they will actually aggravate the condition in the long-term simply because the liver is the most common organ out of sync with these patients. Of course this pattern may not exist in every patient, but it is the most common.

A person may be born with a tendency to develop yang excess or it might be acquired through life. Improper lifestyle habits, poor dietary choices, or disturbed emotions can damage qi and disrupt qi flow. In the diagnosis and treatment of migraines, yang excess and blood stasis are very important concepts. Blood stasis causes a sharp stabbing type of pain, while yang excess causes many disorders in the head.

In clinic every patient may present with a different pattern, or usually a combination of patterns, because every patient is different. Even for one patient, depending on the development of the disease, lifestyle modifications adopted, or environmental changes, the diagnosis will also have to be modified and refined at each specific stage.

3. Organ Manifestation Theory

Organ manifestation theory explains that internal organs have correspondences with sense organs. It is said that the qi of the liver is reflected in the eyes, the qi of the kidney in the ears, and so on for the five major yin organs. This may sound strange to many readers. Please remember that the Chinese understanding of organ function is different from the understanding of modern biomedicine. The organs in Chinese medicine have a variety of functions that are connected through a unique naturalistic theory and confirmed by clinical experience. Sometimes translation of the Chinese term can cause confusion. For example, the organ which is commonly translated as "kidney" in English is involved in reproduction and sexual function along with the urinary system.

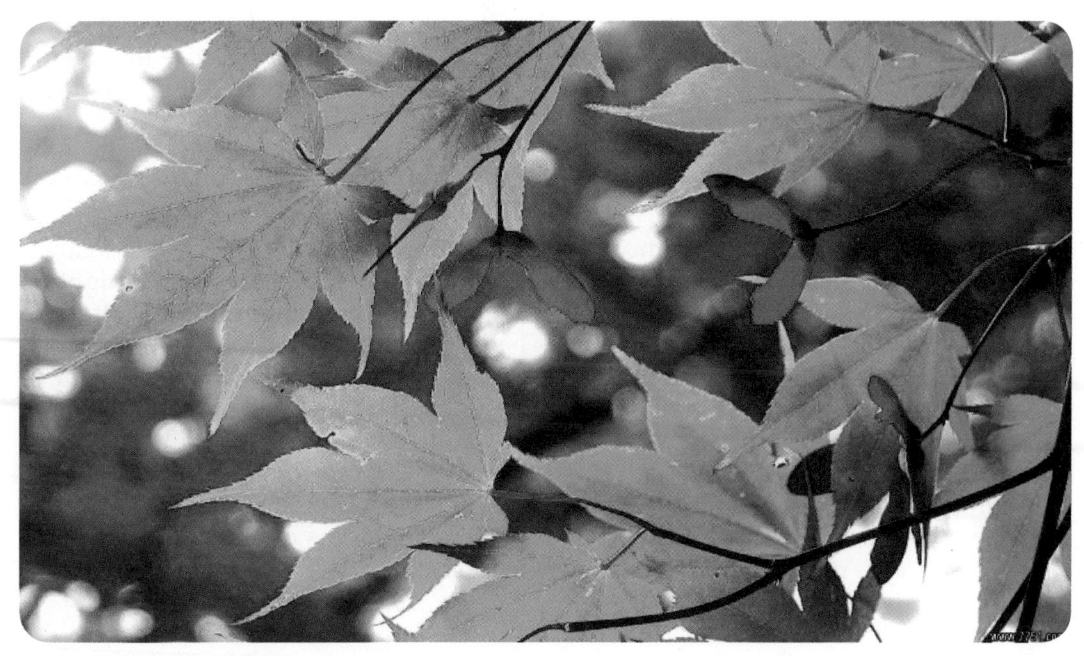

Yin organs include the liver, heart, spleen, lungs and kidneys. The function of the yin organs is to produce, transform, regulate and store fundamental substances such as qi, blood and body fluids. In general, yin organs do not have empty cavities and are therefore called "solid organs".

The six yang organs are made up of the gall bladder, stomach, small intestine, large intestine, bladder and triple burner. The triple burner does not have a physical structure and is considered a functional unit that encompasses the upper, middle, and lower portions of the abdomen and chest. The yang organs are mainly responsible for digesting food and transmitting nutrients to the body. Usually, yang organs are empty cavities so they are termed "hollow organs".

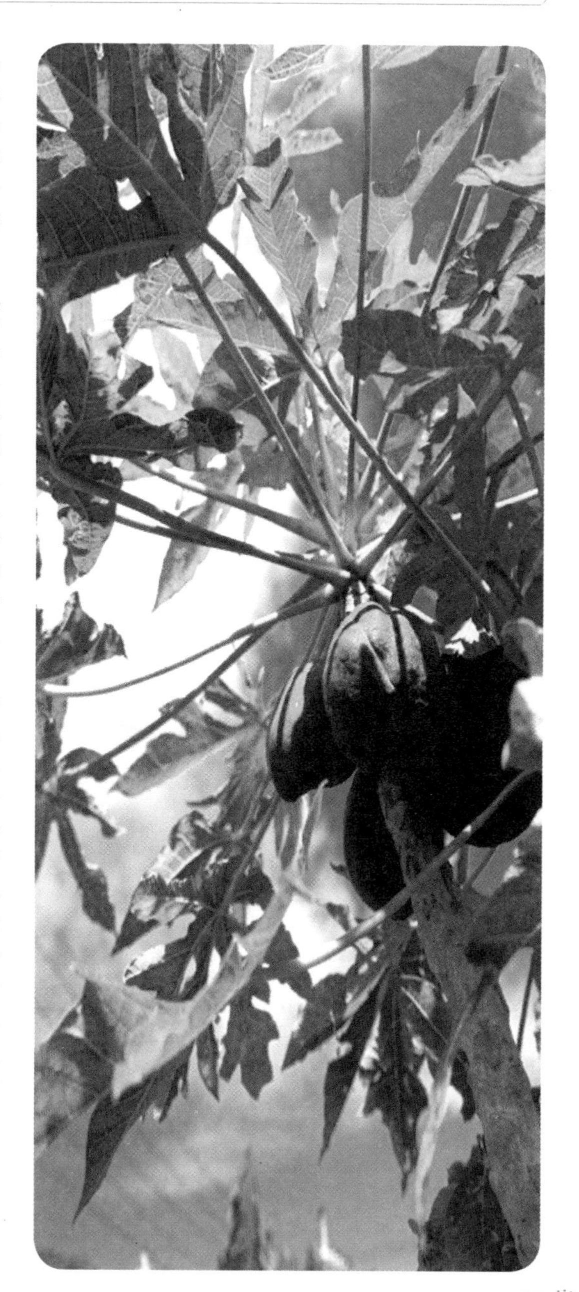

In Chinese medicine, the physiological functions of the body are based on harmonious relationships between yin and yang organs. Central to these relationships is the interior and exterior relationship theory, which states the interior belongs to yin and the exterior belongs to yang. Hence, yin organs are thought to have more internal functions and are called interior organs. They tend to play a more important role in Chinese medical theory and practice. The yang organs, on the other hand, are believed to have more external functions and are therefore considered exterior organs.

After thousands of years of evolution and development, Chinese medicine has stored up a treasure trove of clinical experience. The theories that shape treatment are deeply rooted in practice. This vast clinical experience combined with theory has repeatedly shown strong connections between headaches and internal organ functions. Humans have always had headaches, so information on recognition of the patterns of headache and treatment for these patterns are substantial. Chinese medicine defines headaches according to the pathway of channels they follow. For example, temporal or parietal headaches belong to the gallbladder channel, pain at the top of the head belongs to the liver channel, while forehead pain is associated with the stomach channel, and the back part of the head and neck belong to the urinary bladder channel.

In the clinic, sometimes patients are seen whose migraine pain does not follow usual patterns or channels or exhibits auxiliary complaints. So every situation must be considered carefully and separately, and treated according to the conditions present, often multiple treatment strategies and methods must be used at once. This is accomplished by using pattern differentiation and the concept of holism.

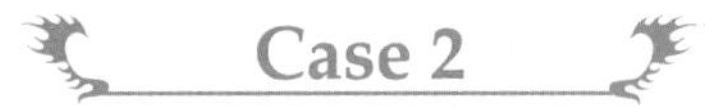

Case 2

Ms. Zhang, 40 years old, visited the out-patient clinic in August, 2006. Before this visit she had been treated for migraines with biomedical pharmaceuticals for many years, but the effects were not consistent, with headaches continuing to occur frequently. Along with her head pain her symptoms included general fatigue and sleep quality so poor it could not relieve this fatigue. The migraine was fixed near both temples and worse at night. This patient's emotions were also severely troubled due to her head pain. She was prone to emotional outbursts and poor temper. Upon examination her tongue appeared pale with dark spots on both sides, with a thin whitish coating. Her pulse was thin, rough, and weak which all indicated bodily weakness accompanied by blood stasis.

An herbal prescription that addressed all the patient's patterns was chosen and the patient was told to come back once a week for re-evaluation and modification of her prescription. Note that it is normal in Chinese medicine for a prescription to be changed weekly or even more frequently, as the patient's condition changes. In just half a month, the general fatigue improved, and the frequency of the migraines lessened. After two months the dosage of the pharmaceuticals she was taking had been gradually reduced. After treatment, all her symptoms had been brought under control, and her quality of life improved accordingly.

Migraine Headaches in Chinese Medicine

The medical literature listed the symptoms of migraine headaches 2,000 years ago in the *Yellow Emperor's Inner Classic,* but it was not until the modern era that it's common occurrence was fully appreciated. Originally migraines were literally called "head wind" in Chinese, and at that time the ancient physicians did not directly distinguish between migraines and other types of headache. Instead, they recorded characteristics of different disease mechanisms, this being the beginning of pattern differentiation. Over several hundred years, accumulated volumes of experience and many well-tested herbal prescriptions emerged. One such herbal formula by a doctor named Wang Qing-ren (1768 C.E. – 1831 C.E.) is called *Orifice-opening Blood-quickening Decoction* which is still commonly used today, 200 years after it's creation.

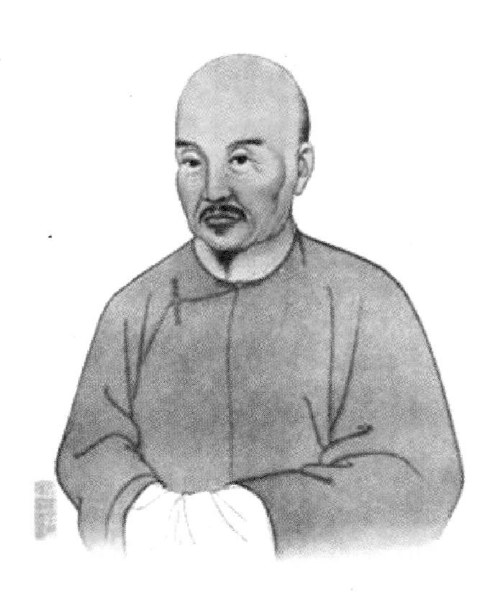

Wang Qing-ren

Over the centuries Chinese medicine's understanding of migraines has developed. With modern recognition of migraine headaches, practitioners of Chinese medicine are able to diagnose the disease based on very specific criteria. Chinese medicine understands that the causes and nature of migraines are complicated. After analyzing thousands of migraine cases, the mechanisms that cause migraines are summed up as follows:

1. Headache Caused By Wind

Recognizing external pathogenic factors is very important in understanding disease development. Biomedicine holds to bacteria, virus and other exogenous factors as the main causes of disease. While Chinese medicine today clearly recognizes these threats, Chinese medicine tradition-

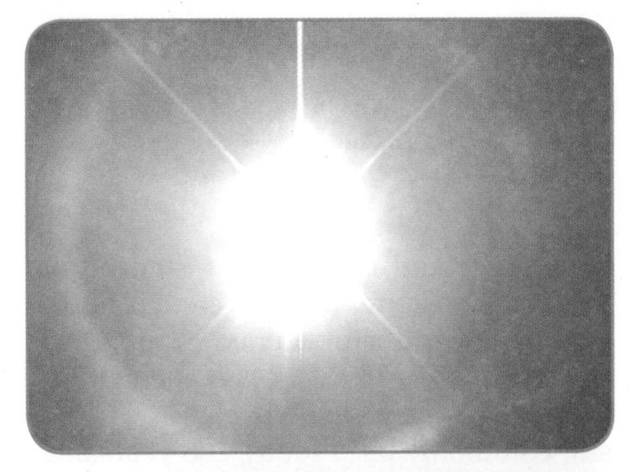

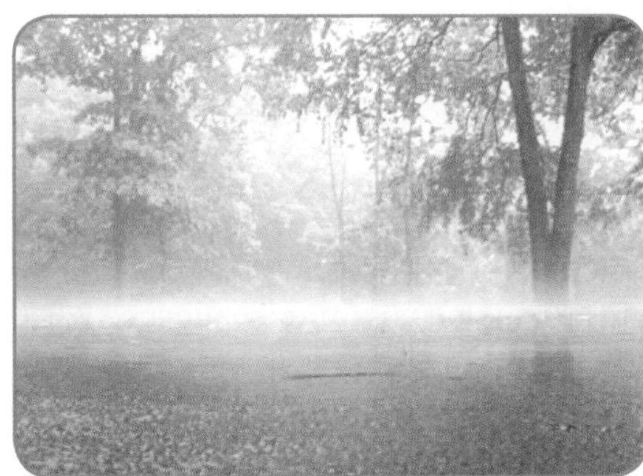

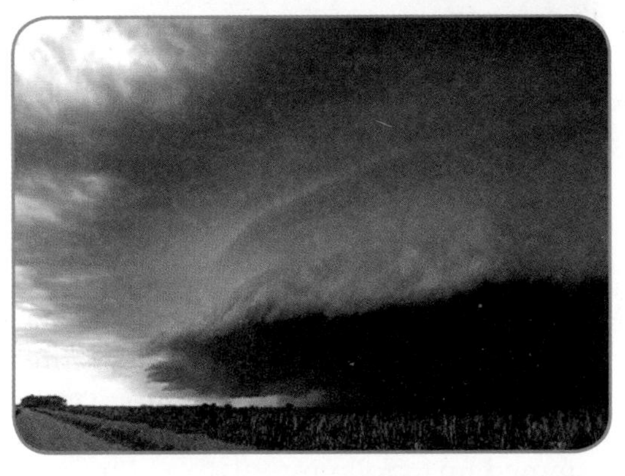

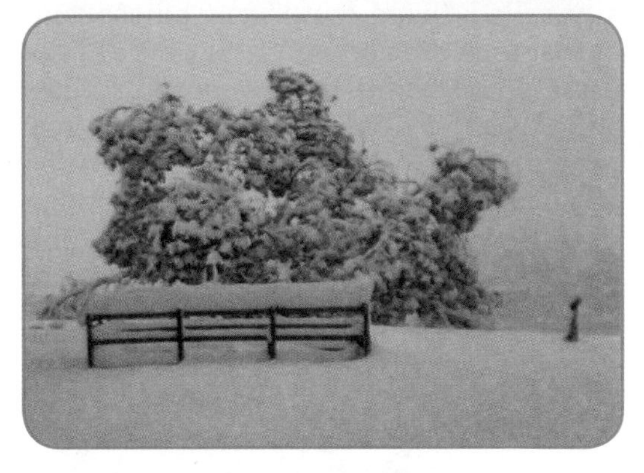

ally recognizes the six external evils that were discussed above as a primary cause of disease. Again, these are: wind, cold, summer-heat, dampness, dryness and fire. If any of these six factors are in excess in the environment, the human body is vulnerable to disease. Furthermore, someone who is weakened is susceptible to invasion, even if the climate is normal. Of these six characteristics, wind is the most varied and complex, just as it is in nature. In the environment the other five factors are fairly straightforward, but wind could be a gentle breeze, a howling gale or a typhoon. It may spin into a tornado, create waves on water or blow every last leaf off of a tree. Wind is unpredictable. Migraines that are caused by wind arrive with a sudden onset, as if blown in like a storm; the pain may move from one part of the head to another, as though propelled by something. Wind in the body has an ascending action, and because of this it tends to rise to the head. Thus migraines and most non-injury head pain are associated with wind.

2. Headache Caused By Deficiency

As mentioned earlier, headaches are labeled according to their particular channel pathway. Pain arising from the temples is different from that starting at the base of the skull or forehead. A deficiency of blood or qi in a certain channel allows wind to enter it, causing disruption of normal qi flow. When the protective qi is not strong, this will also allow an invasion of wind. External factors are always present in life. Indeed, bacteria are everywhere but people don't become sick every day. On the contrary, it is the underlying strength and balance within us that often determines if an external evil is be able to invade the body. Migraines due to deficiency may have a slower onset and may be less severe, but they often linger.

3. Headache Caused By Blood Stasis

Headaches due to blood stasis often present with stabbing pain, prickling pain and other types of heaviness in the head. By identifying the channel affected, the practitioner knows where to direct treatment. But treatment is not decided only by the type and location of pain. Other signs and symptoms are looked for to confirm the diagnosis. For example, a patient with sharp stabbing pain will often show a tongue that is purplish or darker in color with small red spots, and their pulse may be tense or what Chinese medicine calls wiry. These signs confirm blood stasis. If the stabbing pain is on top of the head, it involves the liver channel, whereas in the temples it is the gallbladder channel. Blood stagnation is one of the most frequent patterns present in migraines.

4. Headache Caused By Dampness

Some migraine patients complain of dizziness, lack of appetite, nausea, even vomiting. This is attributed to an accumulation of dampness in the body. The pain may have more of a heavy quality as though the person was wearing a helmet or band wrapped extremely tight around the head. This may also be the cause of migraines that occur before a woman's period. Menstrual migraines commonly combine with abdominal bloating as well. This problem is an imbalance between the liver and spleen. The liver qi flares upward out of control, thus blocking the spleen's ability to transport essence. When this happens, food is not properly digested, and accumulates in the body as dampness, causing appetite problems and bloating.

When treating migraines it is imperative to remember that migraine headaches are a chronic disease, so the duration of therapy will also take time. Expect at least one month of continued therapy. After prolonged treatment, the body's qi may become seriously deficient, if it was not already that way to begin with. Because many of the medicinals used to treat migraines have strong blood moving and wind expelling properties which may damage qi, the body must be nourished when the condition is under control. A normal patient's pattern will not be as simple as those listed above, it will often have multiple facets. The pattern of an individual patient is often mixed with other underlying conditions.

These four causes can cause numerous patterns in the body. However, there are four patters that effectively cover most migraine patients. The signs and symptoms of each pattern are listed in the table below. See if you can identify with one or more of these patterns.

Pattern	Signs and Symptoms
Headache caused by wind	Headaches are varied and complex, unpredictable, often accompanied of a feeling of energy rising to the head
Headache caused by deficiency	Slower onset, less severe, but these kinds of headaches often linger
Headache caused by blood stasis	Characterized by stabbing pain, prickling pain, and heaviness in the head
Headache caused by dampness	Accompanied by dizziness, lack of appetite, nausea, vomiting, and a feeling of wearing a helmet or a band wrapped tightly around the head

Biomedicine has provided all medical practitioners with a more detailed picture of migraine headaches. The treatment of migraines using Chinese medicine has been developing over thousands of years. Its methods and theories are not fixed or stagnant and will continue to develop over time. With the aid of modern technology, Chinese medicine practitioners are able to understand the problems using a combination of their sophisticated philosophy with the latest technological tools and the use of lab tests. The latest guidelines for the treatment of migraine headaches with Chinese medicine provide information on pattern identification, recommended treatment protocols, and treatment evaluation standards.

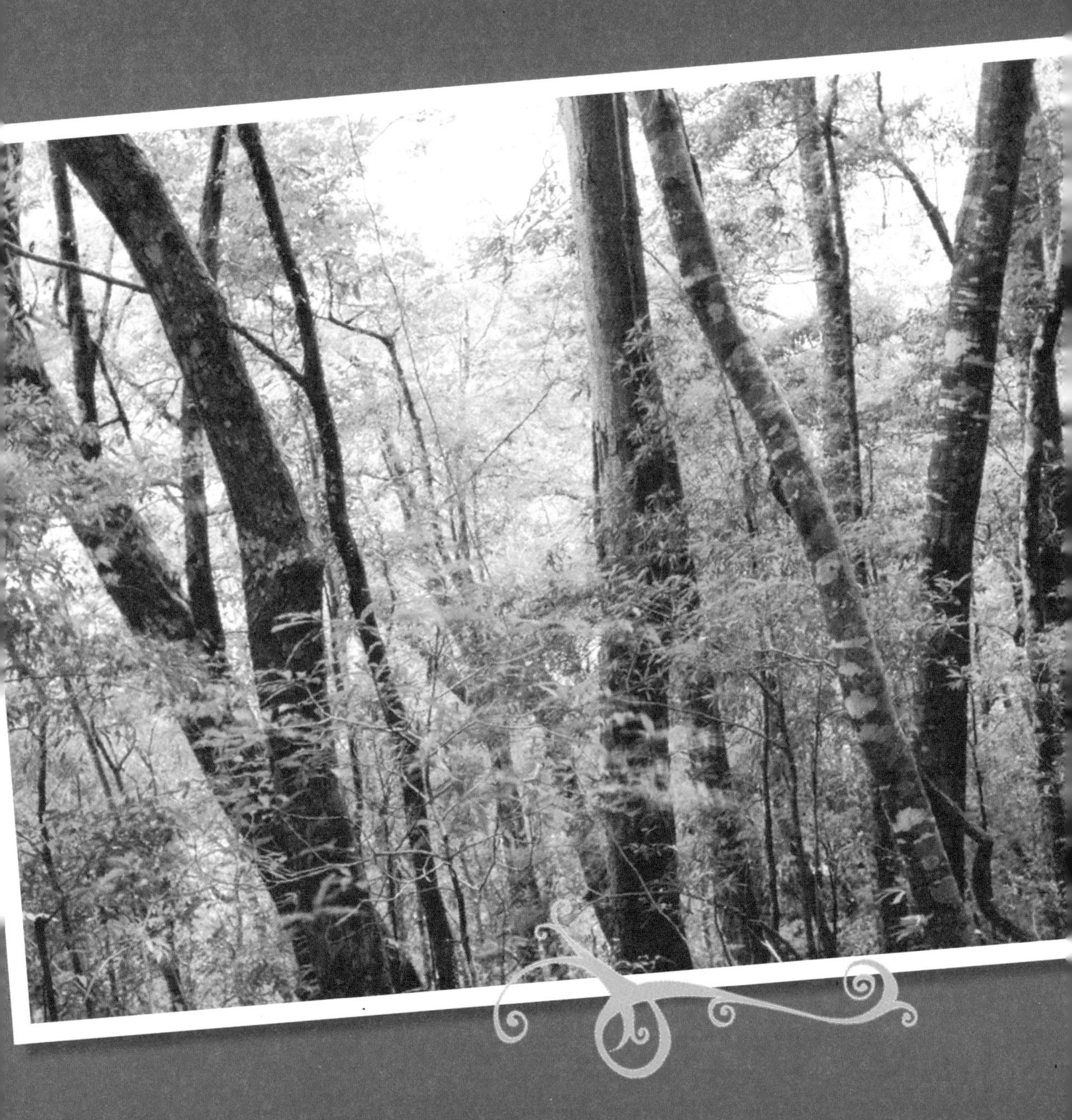

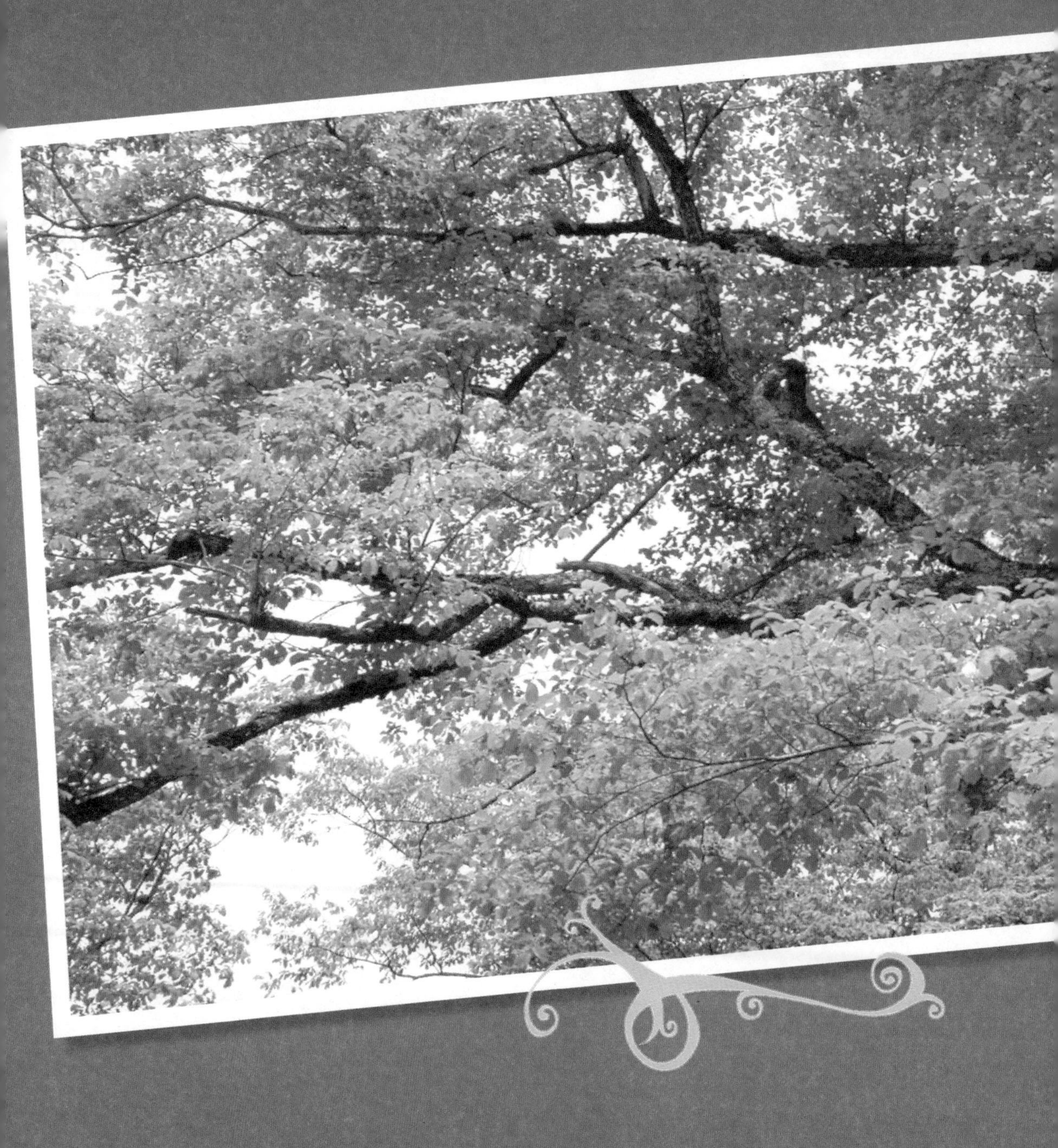

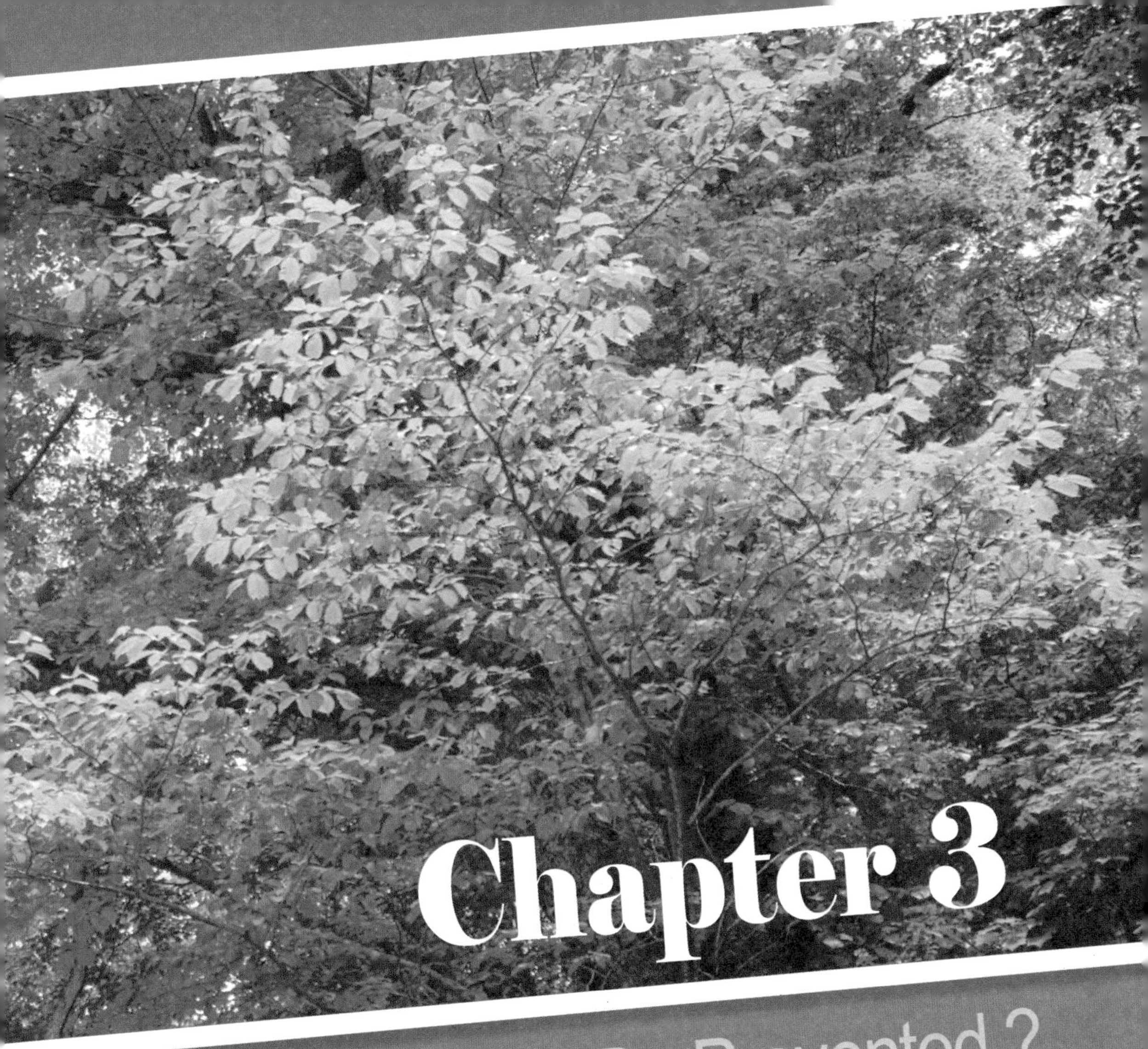

Chapter 3

How Can Migraines Be Prevented ?

So how can one maintain a balance of yin, yang, qi and blood in daily life?

As previously explained, all natural phenomena have yin and yang aspects, and health depends on the balance of yin, yang, qi and blood in the body. Furthermore, there is a constant interaction between the human body and the natural environment. This complex equilibrium is easily affected by the food you eat, your lifestyle choices, the amount of exercise and rest you get, and how you manage your emotions. Your genetic predisposition also plays a role. If you tend to be yang, qi or blood deficient, you can supplement yang, qi or blood by eating foods that promote these substances or by doing exercises that boost yang, qi and blood.

Though Chinese medicine stresses the importance of a peaceful mind for the prevention of disease, the maintenance of psychological health is beyond the scope of this book. Emotional extremes most often lead to qi stagnation which will eventually cause blood stagnation. Maintaining a balanced diet and getting regular exercise will go a long way toward maintaining a calm mind.

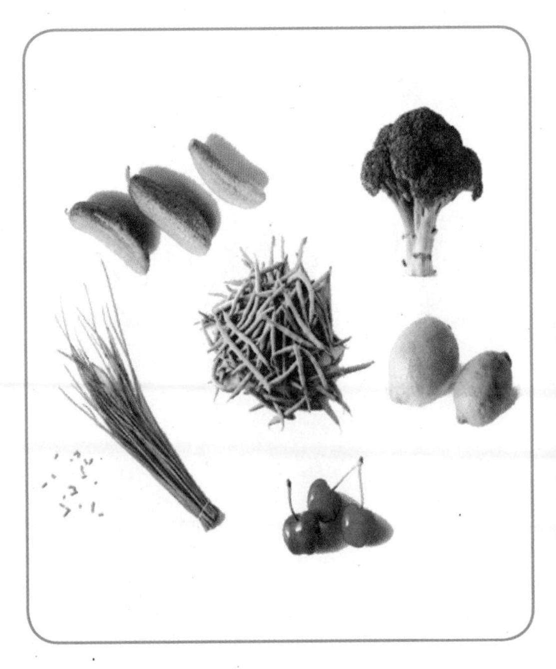

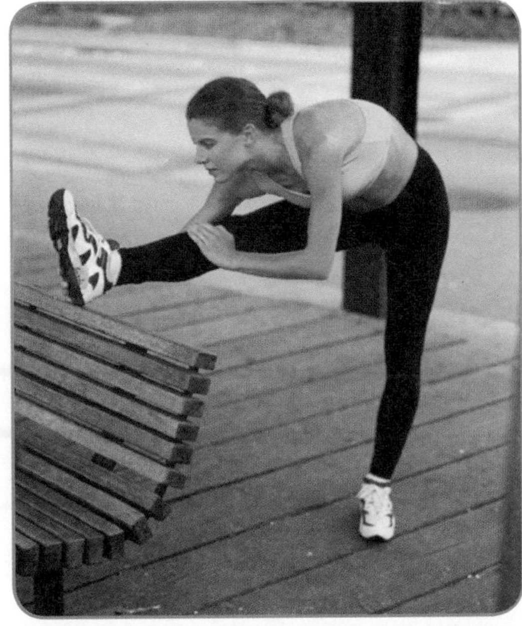

Diet

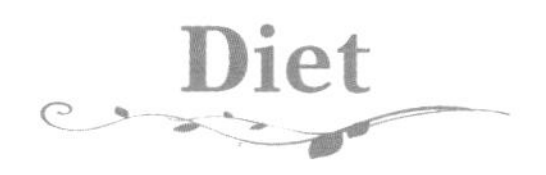

Let food be your medicine and medicine be your food.
-Hippocrates

1. Essentials of Dietary Theory

Dietary therapy is essential to the treatment of migraines according to Chinese medicine. Without proper management of your diet, some medication won't work properly. Chinese medicine holds that food is the best medicine. The things we eat are natural substances that have their own unique qi (properties) just like Chinese medicinals. The properties of Chinese medicinals are used to correct any imbalance of qi, blood, yin, or yang. The properties of food can be used in a similar way. As much as possible, it is better to use food as medicine rather than taking any kind of medication, be it Chinese medicinals or pharmaceuticals. Eating is the most convenient, economic, and delicious prescription a doctor can administer.

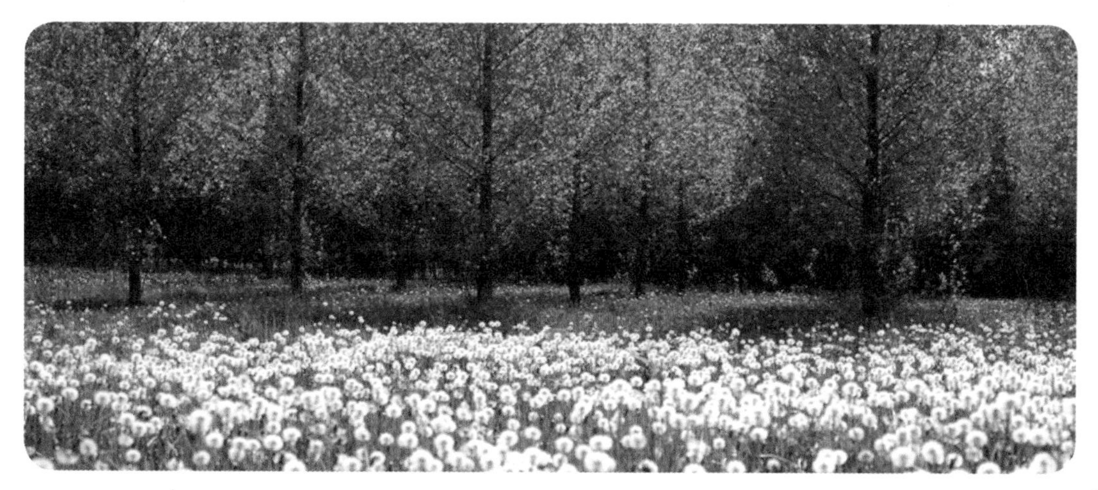

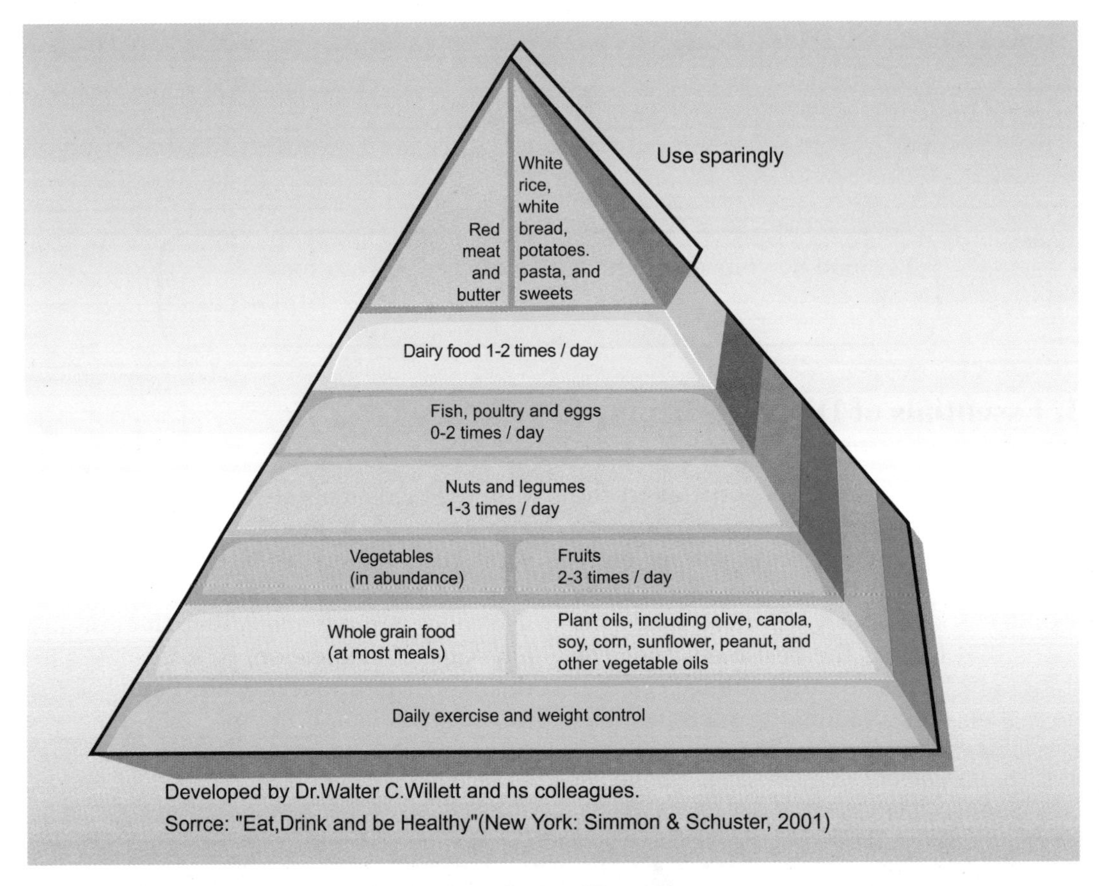

Alternative Food Pyramid

Chinese dietary theory is based on the same principles as herbal medicine. Each food has its own property and is selected based on the patient's pattern to treat disease or preserve health. Biomedical nutritional therapy separates food by content: carbohydrates, protein, fat, vitamins, etc. Chinese medicine concentrates on the qualities of each food item, dividing foods into the categories of taste and temperature. As an example, while the different types of grains are often placed in the same category due to their high carbohydrate content, Chinese medicine, while also recognizing familiar food categories like grains, meat, vegetables, etc., also divides grains into different categories based on their temperature and taste.

Looking at food from the Chinese perspective, beef, onions, and walnuts are all considered warm. Biomedicine on the other hand, would find little in common with these three foods. With the combination of modern nutrition and Chinese dietary theory, food therapy can be very effective.

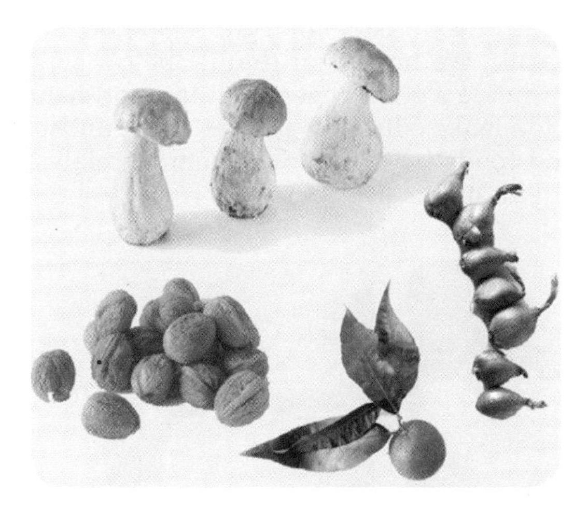

According to Chinese medical theory, each food item can be categorized as having one of the four qi qualities (hot, warm, cool, and cold) and one or more of the five flavors (sour, bitter, sweet, spicy, and salty). This classification of foods follows the same criteria used for medicinals and the application of foods follows the same diagnostic principles and procedures as well. Foods act on the internal organs and influence the qi of the body, which can be used to preserve health and treat disease. The main difference between food and medicinal substances is that food is generally milder when compared with Chinese medicinals. That's why food is taken daily and medicinals only when necessary.

To eat a balanced diet, in terms of Chinese medicine, is to balance the qi of the food. A diet too lopsided in one direction or the other for too long will eventually cause an imbalance of qi, blood, yin and/or yang. For those already suffering from disease, special foods are chosen based on the patient's individual condition. Dietary prescriptions in Chinese medicine are made according to pattern identification. Biomedicine calculates the calories, vitamins, fat content, etc. precisely. When combined, the migraine patient can have a very well-designed dietary regimen.

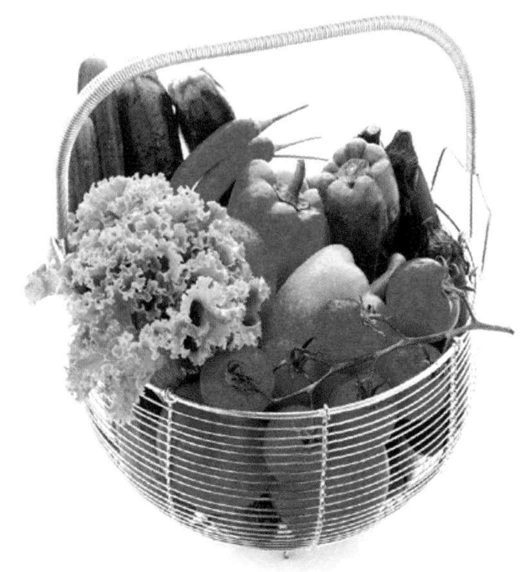

Properly chosen, food can be used as medicine. Some Chinese medicinals can be used as food and added into your diet. Indeed, many common spices (like cinnamon, cardamom, ginger, garlic) are commonly used in herbal treatment. In Chinese medicine, the line between food and medicine is a blurry one. Hot food like peppers and chilies has a warming effect on the body, while cold food like tomatoes and bananas can cool the body. Neutral food doesn't have much influence on the body, and are an important part of maintaining a healthy balance. For example, rice is neutral and thus can be consumed daily, providing nourishment while not having a drastic effect on the body's function.

The following table is an example of some common food items and their properties. A complete list of the properties of food is beyond the scope of this book. We hope that the list below will provide a good general outline, and help you make educated guesses about unlisted foods by comparing them to related items on the list.

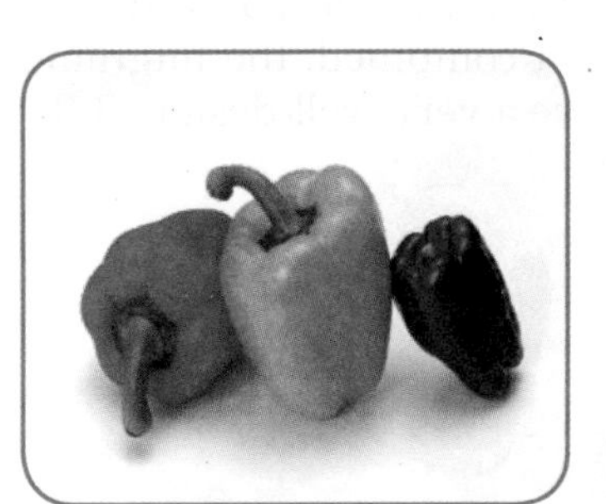

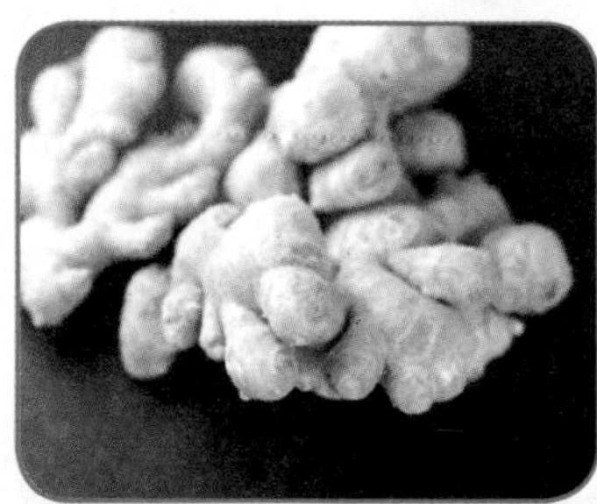

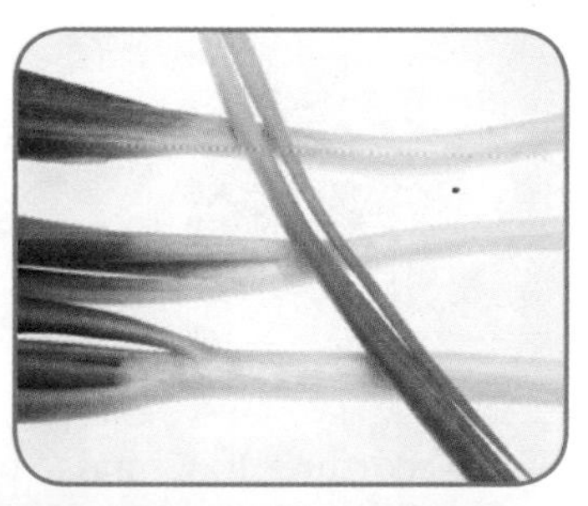

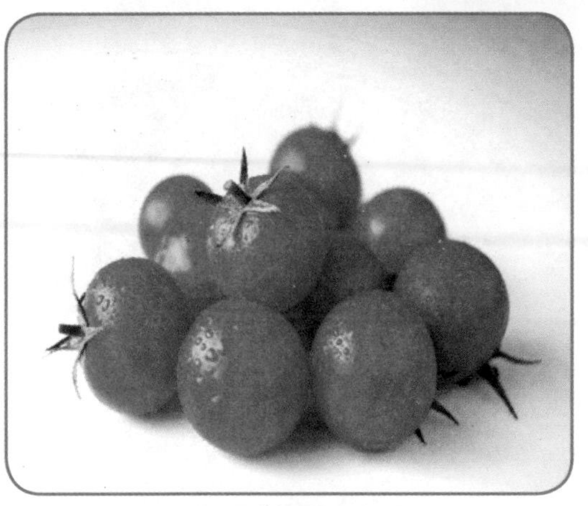

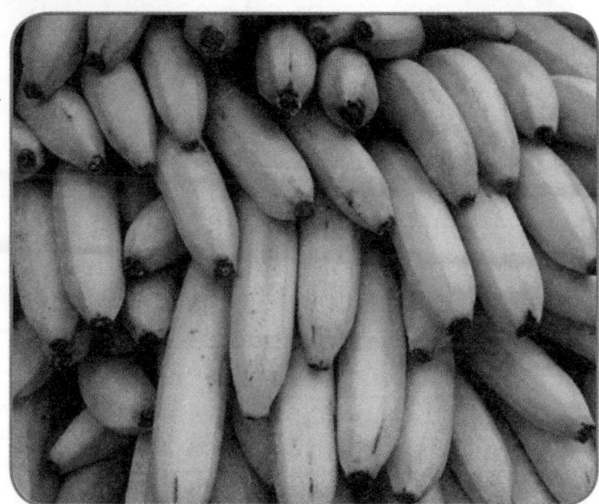

Common Food and Their Properties

Category	Hot	Warm	Neutral	Cold	Cool
Function	Increase yang, move qi, warm the body	Strengthen yang, warm qi and the organs	Build qi and body fluids. Harmonize the body	Cool heat. Calm the spirit	Slow down qi, clear heat, and nourish fluids
Beverages	Alcohol	Cocoa, Coffee, Wine		Water	Black tea, Fruit juices, Peppermint tea, Soy milk
Condiments			Honey	Salt, Soy sauce	
Dairy		Butter, Goat cheese	Cheese	Cow's milk	Yogurt
Animal products	Lamb	Beef, Chicken, Eel, Salmon	Carp, Duck, Eggs, Pork, Goose	Shrimp, Crayfish	Rabbit
Fruits and vegetables		Cherry, Fennel, Leek, Peach, Onion	Carro, Cauli flower, Grape, Fig, Plum, Potato	Asparagus, Banana, Orange, Rhubarb, Seaweed, Tomato, Watermelon	Celery, Cucumber, Soy bean, Sprouts, Spinach, Zucchini
Grains and legumes			Corn, Lentil, Millet, Peas, Rice, Spelt		Barley, Tofu, Wheat
Herbs and spices	Cinnamon, Chili, Curry, Garlic, Ginger, Paprika, Pepper	Anise, Basil, Rosemary		Dandelion, Yellow gentian	Tarragon
Nuts		Walnut	Hazelnut		

(The table is adapted from P23, Joweh Kastner. *Chinese Nutrition Therapy*. Thieme Stuttgart, New York, 2004)

2. Migraine Food Triggers

Twenty percent of migraine headaches occur after a meal according to the latest survey by American medical specialists. These are migraines caused by food triggers. These kinds of headaches are caused by the chemical composition of some kinds of food, which when consumed lead to a dilation of cerebral blood vessels in susceptible people and cause migraine symptoms[13].

Some medical specialists suggest those who suffer from migraines without knowing the causes should keep a record: the time of migraine onset and the diet before it. The following foods are commonly seen to initiate a headache: chocolate, cheese, smoked sausage and meat (also some dried fruits), nuts (such as walnut, filbert), oranges, lemons, plum, salted fish, foods with color additives and preservative, and alcohol, especially red wine and beer[6].

Food to avoid

★ Three items to avoid

Cheese, chocolate and citrus fruit. These contain tyrosine which can cause blood vessel spasms. In addition, pickled sardines, chicken liver, tomato, milk and other drinks with lactic acid should all be avoided.

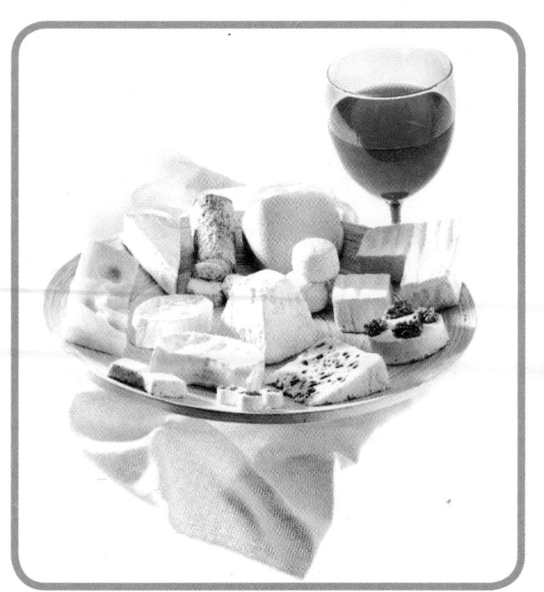

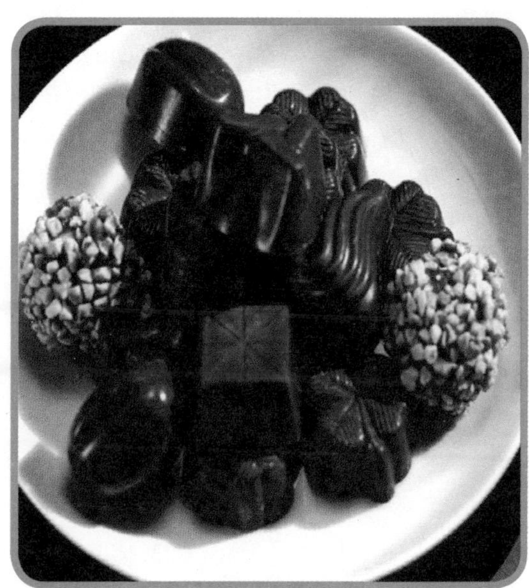

★ **Sausages and hot dogs**

Pickled and processed meat, such as sausages, hot dogs, ham and cured meats contain nitrites and often MSG (mono-sodium glutamate). These chemicals and these kinds of food can aggravate headaches.

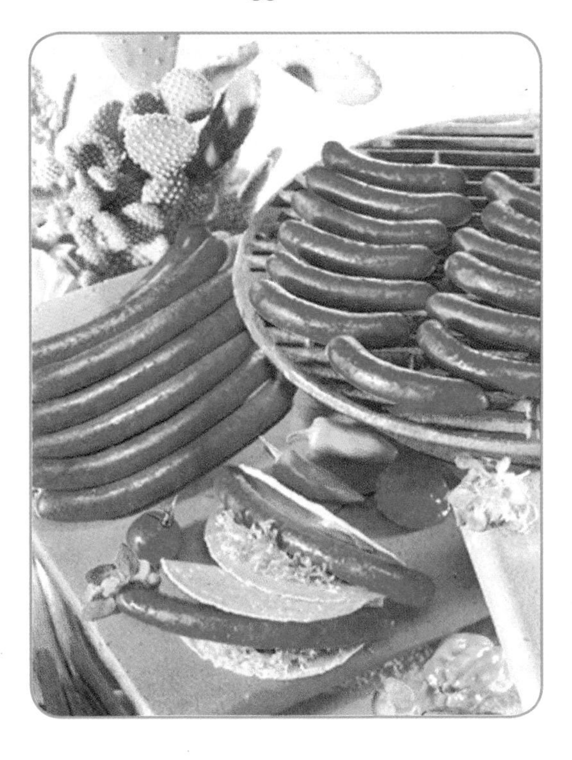

★ **Sugar substitutes**

Some researchers have learned that sugar substitutes such as aspartame can irritate nerve terminals and increase muscle tension. This increased tension and imbalance may lead to more migraines. Beware of products which list "Amino acids", "Aspartic acid" or "Phenylalanine". These should also be avoided. For those with sugar sensitivities, it is better to use a natural substance such as honey instead of artificial sweetener.

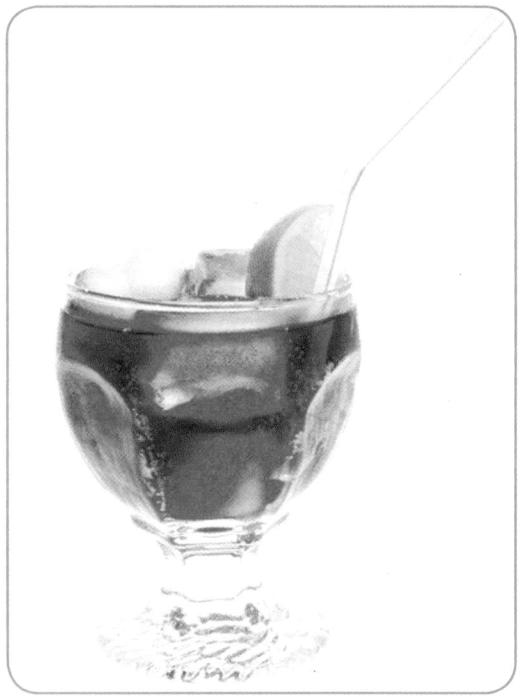

★ **Red wine**

All kinds of alcohol can induce migraine headaches, especially red wine, which contains many chemicals that can potentially induce a headache. For those prone to headaches, if you want to drink, then vodka or distilled spirits should be selected over wine.

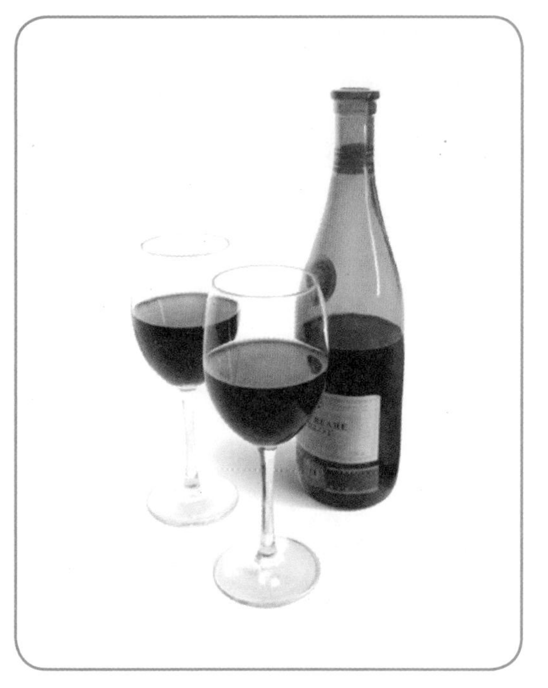

★ **Coffee**

Caffeine can stimulate the nervous system and cause sleep disorders. Those who drink it often (daily) can easily become addicted. If the person stops the consumption, intense headaches can occur during withdrawal. This is a clear lesson that common substances can have strong effects on our nervous systems. It is best to drink only one cup of coffee or less per day.

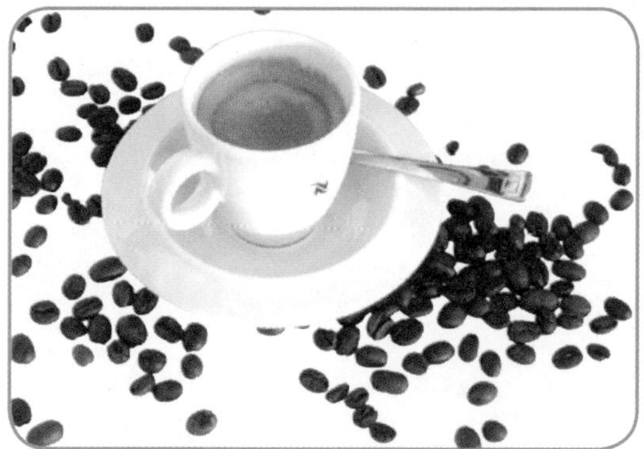

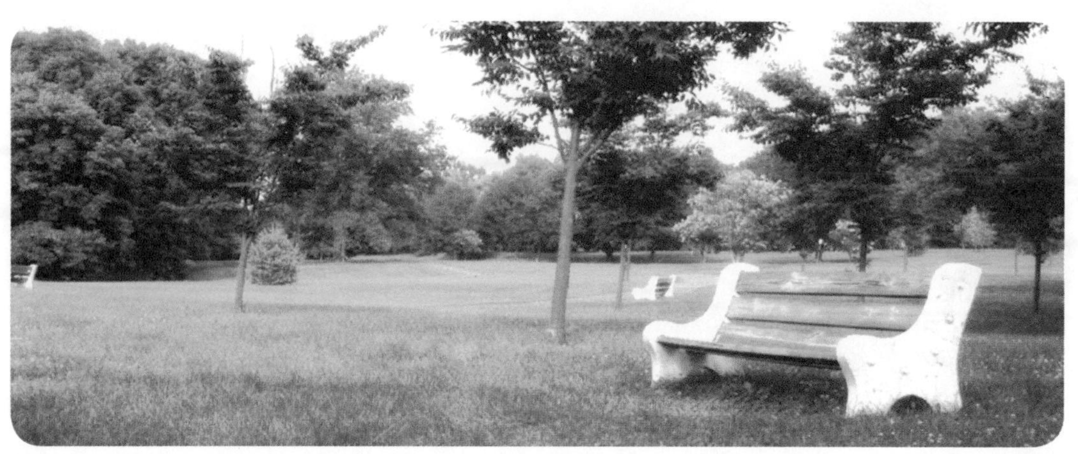

3. Special Items for Migraines

The following items which are highly recommended by Chinese medicine practitioners for patients with migraines. Some of these foods are not common to the Western diet, but because they are so helpful in reducing the frequency and intensity of migraine headaches, patients are strongly advised to find these wonderful foods and integrate them into their diets.

Cereal grains

Cereal grains contain high amounts of the mineral magnesium, which can adjust blood flow and help relax muscle tissue. Migraine headaches can arise in some people if magnesium content is below normal. To prevent this, a person should get approximately 500 - 750 mg of magnesium daily.

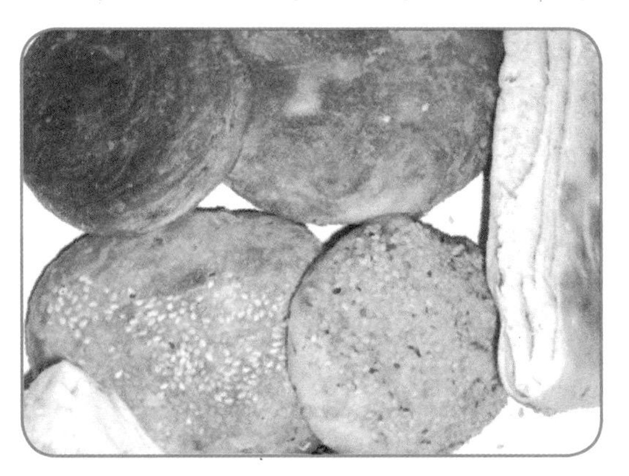

Good food sources for magnesium include millet, corn, sunflower seeds, apricot seeds, cashew and hazelnut, cabbage or mustard greens, snake butter mushrooms, laver (a type of seaweed), peaches, longan fruit, walnuts and peanuts.

Starches

This kind of food, also known as amylaceous food, includes cooked rice, potatoes, biscuits and bread. Although wheat can induce migraines for those with wheat sensitivities, for those who can tolerate it, wheat and other starchy food may actually help to relieve pain. Some research has shown that starchy food can relieve head pain, nausea, and even shorten the duration of migraines. By trying various kinds of amylaceous food, your own experience will tell you if it is effective for your migraines.

Fish

Fish and fish oil have been shown to reduce migraine frequency. You may try

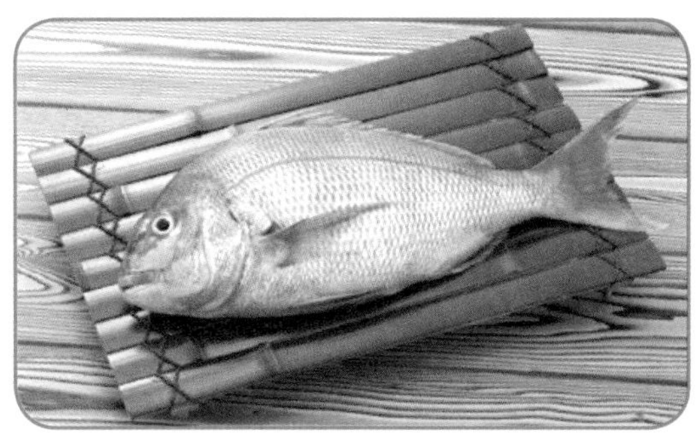

eating fish three times per week, or taking fish oil as a dietary supplement.

Green tea

Chinese people long ago discovered the healing properties of tea leaves and have used them as herbal medicine for generations. For example, people added tea leaves to their food to supply nutrients or as an antidote to environmental toxins. It was not until the Han dynasty (206 B.C.E. - 220 C.E.), that methods of preparing tea became more standardized and tea became a drink whose popularity rivaled wine.

Green tea leaves are freshly picked and only go through a process of heating and drying, not fermentation. This enables the leaves to keep their original green color and retain more natural substances like polyphenols, fluoride and chlorophyll. This kind of tea is produced all over China and is the most popular type of tea. Two popular varieties are Dragon Well (*Long Jing*) from Zhejiang Province, and *Bi Luo Chun* from Jiangsu Province.

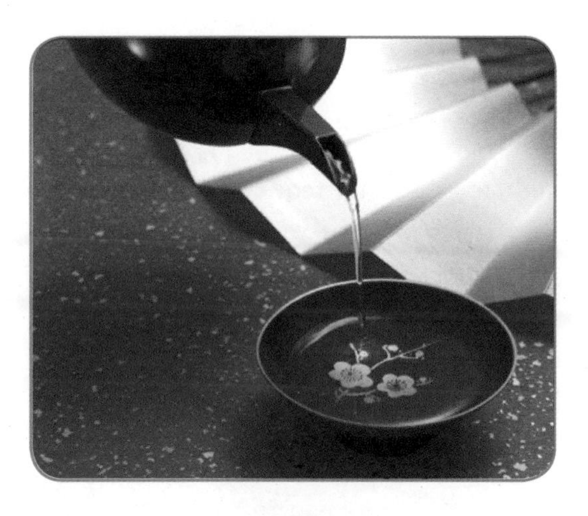

According to Chinese medicine's understanding, tea has both sweet and bitter flavors and possesses cooling properties. Tea helps to refresh the mind, enhance alertness and boost concentration. Tea can also promote the production of body fluids, quench thirst, clear heat, resolve phlegm, and promote digestion and urination. Below are two tea recipes that may not be so well known in the West.

Chrysanthemum tea

Use 2 g of green tea plus a few dried white chrysanthemum flowers. Both are steeped in a pot of hot water for five minutes. This blend cleanses the liver, benefits the eyes and is good for those with hypertension, blurred vision and headaches.

Fresh plum tea

Using 10 - 150 g of fresh plums, boil them with 320 ml of water for three minutes, then add 2 g green tea, 25 g honey, bring to a boil, and steep for a few minutes. This tea clears heat, drains dampness, benefits the liver and relieves stress.

4. Everyday Eating

Below are some suggestions on medicinal ingredients that can be used in simple recipes plus common foods that are good for migraine headaches. Most of the medicinals are best used in soups and stews, though more specific cooking information is listed in the recipes. We hope that with the advice of your practitioner, you can learn which recipes and ingredients are right for you and incorporate them into your daily routine. You should be able to buy the necessary ingredients in small amounts to be used in cooking from you practitioner, online or in an Asian supermarket.

The amounts given are in grams and liters. To convert to ounces and cups, 30 grams is roughly equal to one ounce, and one liter is about four cups.

Recipes for different patterns

☆ Migraine headaches due to wind-cold

Signs and Symptoms: a headache that starts after being exposed to wind and cold. The pain is often situated along the neck and back. This person often feels an aversion to wind and/or cold, and likes to wrap their head and neck in cloth or a hat, or lie under a blanket. There may be nasal obstruction, sometimes rhinitis (runny nose), lack of thirst, and the tongue will have a thin white coating.

Rice porridge with onion and prepared soybean

Ingredients: rice 50 - 100 g, scallion white 10 g, prepared soybean 10 g.

To prepare: cook the rice normally in a rice cooker or on the stovetop. Add the cooked rice, scallion white and prepared soybean to 1 - 1.5 liters water. Bring to a boil and simmer until the ingredients are well blended, and the liquid is a thick consistency.

Chuanxiong and dahurian angelica with fish

Ingredients: one Asian carp, or other large fresh water white fish, chuanxiong 3 - 9 g, dahurian angelica 6 - 9 g.

To prepare: Wrap the chuanxiong and Dahurian Angelica in cheesecloth. Add it to the pot with water and the fish. Stew over slow fire until the fish is well done. Flavor with mild seasoning, as the herbs create much flavor of their own.

☆ Migraines due to wind-heat

Signs and Symptoms: The headache is sharp and pounding, eye pressure with flashing light, thirst, possible fever or feeling of heat, aversion to wind, constipation and yellow urine. The tongue will have a yellow coating.

Drink of mulberry leaf, chrysanthemum flower, mint, and bamboo leaf
Ingredients: Mulberry leaf 10 g, bamboo leaf 15 - 30 g, chrysanthemum flower 10 g, and mint 6 g.

To prepare: Rinse the above four herbs. Place them into teapot with boiling water and steep for 10 minutes.

Chuanxiong tea
Ingredients: Chuanxiong 3 g, green tea leaves 6 g.

To prepare: Add chuanxiong and the green tea leaves with enough water to cover them by 3 cm (1 in.). Bring to a boil, reduce heat and simmer for 20 minutes. Drink it warm.

☆ Migraines due to hyperactive liver-yang

Signs and Symptoms: Headache with dizziness and possible muscle tics, irritability, insomnia or dream-disturbed sleep, bitter taste in the mouth, and occasional flank or rib side pain. The tongue will be red with a thin yellow coat.

Gastrodia and carp
Ingredients: Gastrodia 25 g, chuanxiong 10 g, poria 10 g, one fresh carp (about 1000 g).

To prepare: Cut chuanxiong and poria into small pieces, and put them together with the gastrodia into water that has been used to wash rice and soak for 4 - 6 hours. Next, take out the gastrodia and place it on top of rice to be steamed after cutting it into smaller pieces. When the rice is cooked through, stuff the fish with all three herbs. Add some ginger and green onion and bake the fish for about 30 minutes. When cooked through, the fish and rice can be eaten together. Note: other types of white fish can also be used.

☆ Migraines due to deficient blood

Signs and Symptoms: Chronic headaches and dizziness that are worse when the patient is tired. Fatigue, poor appetite, dull facial expression, heart palpitations, shortness of breath, and dislike of cold. The tongue will be pale.

Chicken with yellow essence
Ingredients: Yellow essence 30 g, codonopsis 30 g, dioscorea 30 g, one chicken (about 500 g).

To prepare: Cut the chicken meat into 3 cm square pieces. Boil in water for 3 minutes. Remove from pot. Place chicken into a steam boiler and add ginger, green onion, salt, and the herbs. Steam cook over medium-low heat for 3 hours.

☆ Migraines due to phlegm

Signs and Symptoms: Headache, dizziness, chest and abdominal distension; nausea, vomiting, loss of appetite. The tongue will be swollen with teeth marks on its edges and have a white greasy coating.

Bamboo shoot porridge

Ingredients: Winter bamboo shoots 100 g, minced pork 50 g, rice 100 g, sesame oil 25 g.

To prepare: Cook the rice normally in a rice cooker or stovetop. While rice is cooking, cut winter bamboo shoots into slivers and heat in sesame oil until browned. In a large skillet, add minced pork, bamboo, and season with green onion, ginger and salt. Cook until meat is done. Combine rice with the sauteed bamboo and meat and 2 - 6 cups water. Heat together and serve.

Pinellia and dioscorea porridge

Ingredients: Dioscorea 30 g, prepared pinellia 30 g.

To prepare: Crush the pinellia and add to a pot with 6 cups of water. Bring to a boil and simmer for 30 minutes. Grind dioscorea into powder and add to the pinellia decoction. Boil again, simmering for 20 minutes, then add sugar to taste.

☆ **Migraines due to blood stasis**

Signs and Symptoms: head pain for long duration, fixed in one location with stabbing pain. The tongue may appear purplish or dark with red or dark spots.

Chuanxiong and carthamus tea

Ingredients: Chuanxiong 3 - 6 g, carthamus 3 g, green tea 3 - 6 g.

To prepare: Boil chuanxiong, carthamus and tea with water, drink it like tea.

☆ **Migraines due to kidney deficiency**

Signs and Symptoms: Dull heavy pain, worse if the head is shaken, ringing in the ears, insomnia, memory loss, pain and/or weakness in low back and knees, spermatorrhea. The tongue will be red in color and thin.

Lycium, walnut and chicken soup

Ingredients: Lycium 30 g, walnut 30 g, and 500 g chicken.

To prepare: Boil chicken as if making chicken soup. At the half-way point add lycium fruit, walnut, ginger, green onion and salt. Cook the soup over medium low heat about half an hour.

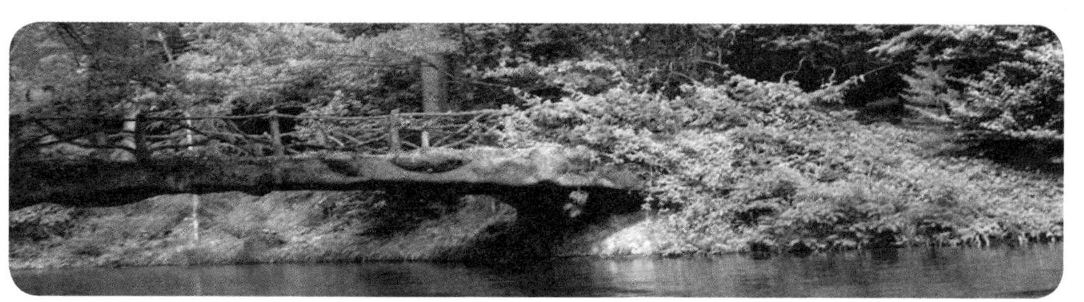

English Name	Chinese Name	Pinyin	Latin Name
Scallion White	葱白	*Cōng bái*	Bulbus Allii Fistulosi
Prepared Soybean	淡豆豉	*Dàn dòu chǐ*	Semen Sojae Praeparatum
Chuanxiong Rhizome	川芎	*Chuān xiōng*	Rhizoma Chuanxiong
Dahurian Angelica Root	白芷	*Bái zhǐ*	Radix Angelicae Dahuricae
Mulberry Leaf	桑叶	*Sāng yè*	Folium Mori
Bamboo Leaf	竹叶	*Zhú yè*	Herba Lophatheri
Chrysanthemum Flower	菊花	*Jú huā*	Flos Chrysanthemi
Imperata Rhizome	白茅根	*Bái máo gēn*	Rhizoma Imperatae
Mint	薄荷	*Bò hé*	Herba Menthae
Gastrodia Rhizome	天麻	*Tiān má*	Rhizoma Gastrodiae
Poria	茯苓	*Fú líng*	Poria
Ginseng Root	人参	*Rén shēn*	Radix et Rhizoma Ginseng
Lycium Fruit	枸杞子	*Gǒu qǐ zǐ*	Fructus Lycii
Ginger Rhizome	生姜	*Shēng jiāng*	Rhizoma Zingiberis Recens
Yellow Essence	黄精	*Huáng jīng*	Rhizoma Polygonati
Codonopsis Root	党参	*Dǎng shēn*	Radix Codonopsis
Dioscorea Rhizome	山药	*Shān yào*	Rhizoma Dioscoreae
Pinellia Rhizome	半夏	*Bàn xià*	Rhizoma Pinelliae
Carthamus Flower	红花	*Hóng huā*	Flos Carthami
Walnut	核桃仁	*Hé táo rén*	Semen Juglandis

Exercise

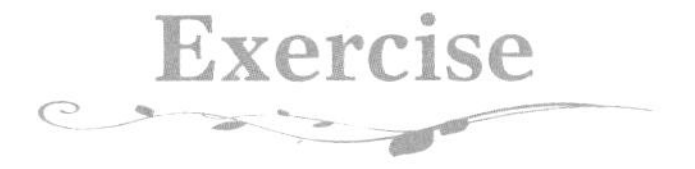

1. What Kinds of Exercise are Helpful?

Physical activity is one of the most beneficial therapies for patients with migraines. Together with medication and proper diet, it is an essential part of successful migraine management. As to what kinds of exercises are appropriate, the first principle is to choose one that won't strain you excessively or make you overly tired. Another equally important principle is to choose one you like. Walking and yoga are good choices. Other good activities are hiking, cycling, swimming, or tai ji. It is not beneficial to exercise to exhaustion. The best time to exercise is in the morning before breakfast or in the evening after dinner. Exercise regularly and consistently for the most benefit.

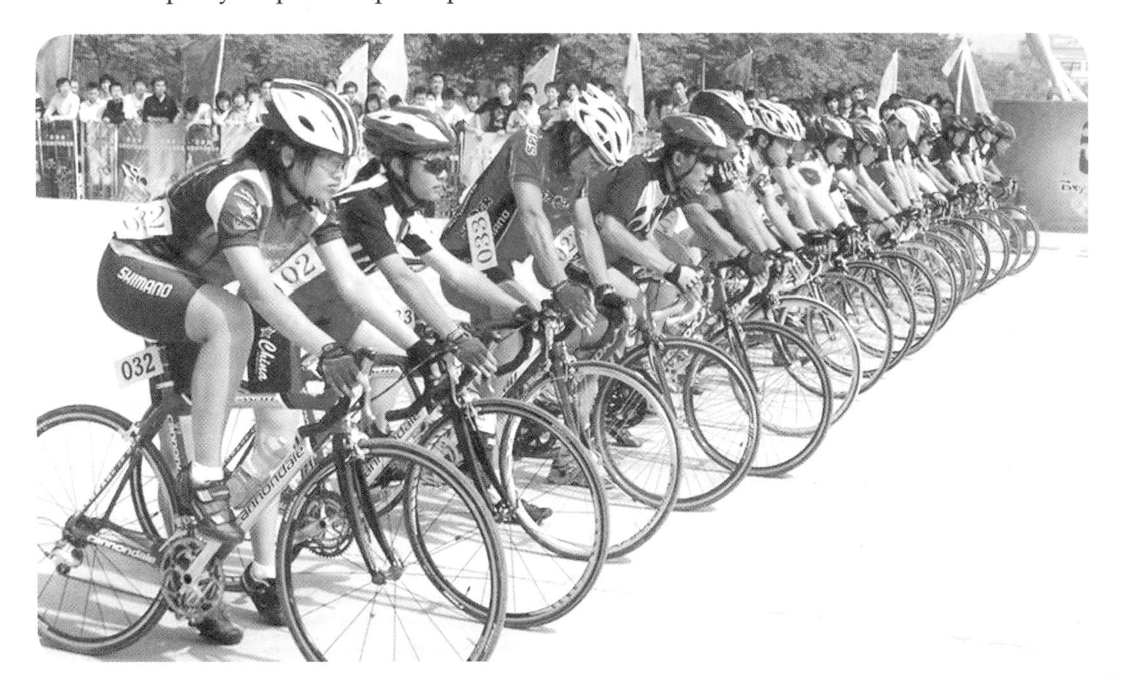

2. Qi Gong and Tai Ji

❶ Tai ji quan

Tai ji quan, a unique body-mind exercise, is a martial art based on Daoist philosophy and yin-yang theory. It is a special kind of kung fu practiced to maintain health and for self-defense. Because it doesn't demand a lot of bodily energy or strength to learn, it is suitable for both young and old, and makes a great aerobic exercise. The more you practice, the better you will understand your own body, helping to coordinate and clear your body and mind. You will feel peace and grace physically, psychologically, and emotionally after practicing tai ji quan. Modern research has shown it to boost immunity, and it can help patients regulate their qi and blood and improve their overall sense of well-being[14-16].

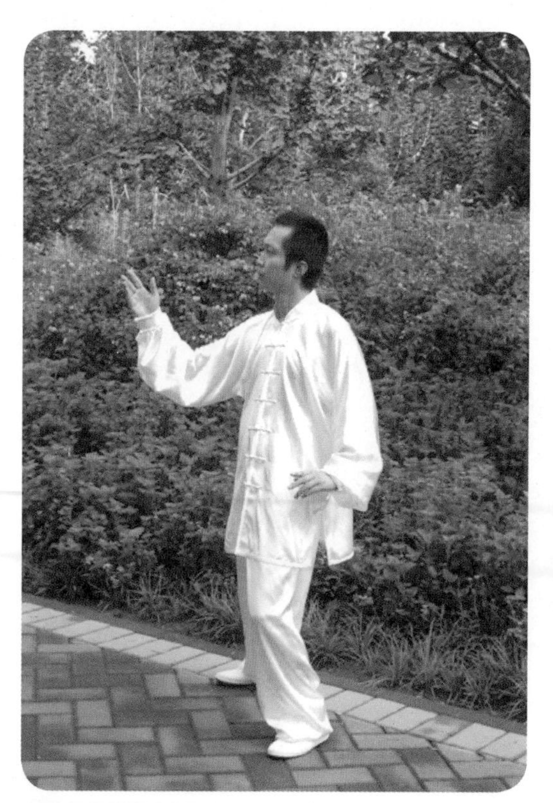

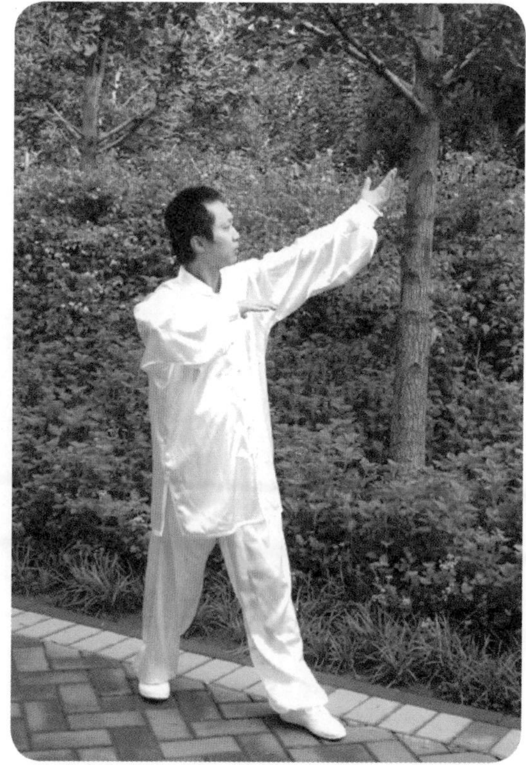

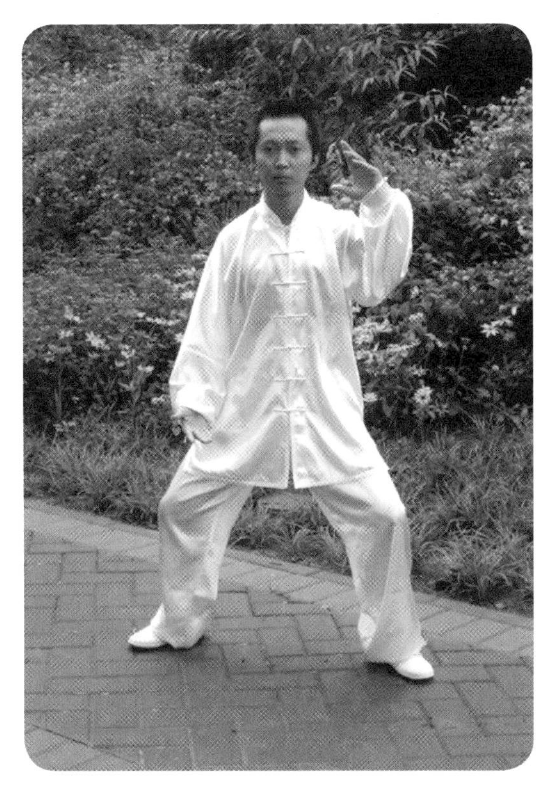

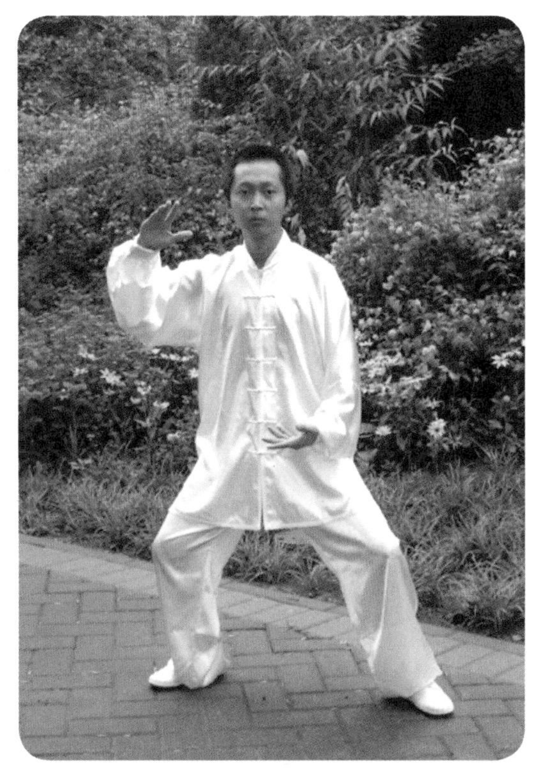

It is not clear when or where tai ji quan first began. There have been many schools during its development over the centuries. Presently, the five major schools are Yang, Chen, Wu, Sun, and Wu. Whatever school you practice, you will be taught similar slow, graceful, smooth movements. The essence of tai ji quan is its harmonious natural movements; representing the constant transformation and interaction of yin and yang. Its movements are simple but subtle. It takes time, discipline and persistence to master the forms.

It is highly recommended that you learn tai ji from a qualified instructor. A book or DVD can help you get a rough idea about the basic movements and the sequence. But tai ji is not dancing or modeling, where the external form is most important; nor is it aerobics where the point is simply to get the heart rate going. You need an experienced instructor to guide you through the internal process as well as the external movements.

- You need to practice on a regular basis. Find a quiet place with fresh air. After you become familiar with the movements you will start to feel the subtle difference it makes on your body.

- With a calm mind, guide your movements consciously, breathing slowly, deeply and naturally. Your movements should be stable, constant, gentle, and fluent.

- Tai ji quan is both yin and yang: moving and still, hard and gentle, backward and forward, flexible and firm. Practicing tai ji can boost your qi and harmonize yin and yang in your body. It can make you feel refreshed and relaxed, and increase your awareness and enthusiasm for life.

By learning to move slowly but consistently, your body can be trained to follow the subtle instructions of the brain. Gradually, coordination between your body and mind will be improved. A practitioner who had been learning tai ji for five years once fell down from a riding bicycle and to her surprise she was not hurt at all. At the instant she fell down, her body naturally folded into the best position to avoid a head injury. This kind of ability to adjust instinctively to the environment reveals a higher level of vitality and leads to a greater state of health. Tai ji is a door into the world of rediscovering your own body and how it relates to the world outside.

② Qi gong

Throughout the history of Chinese medicine, doctors have paid great attention to qi gong and many of them were great masters of qi gong as well. The great doctor Zhang Zhong-jing recommended

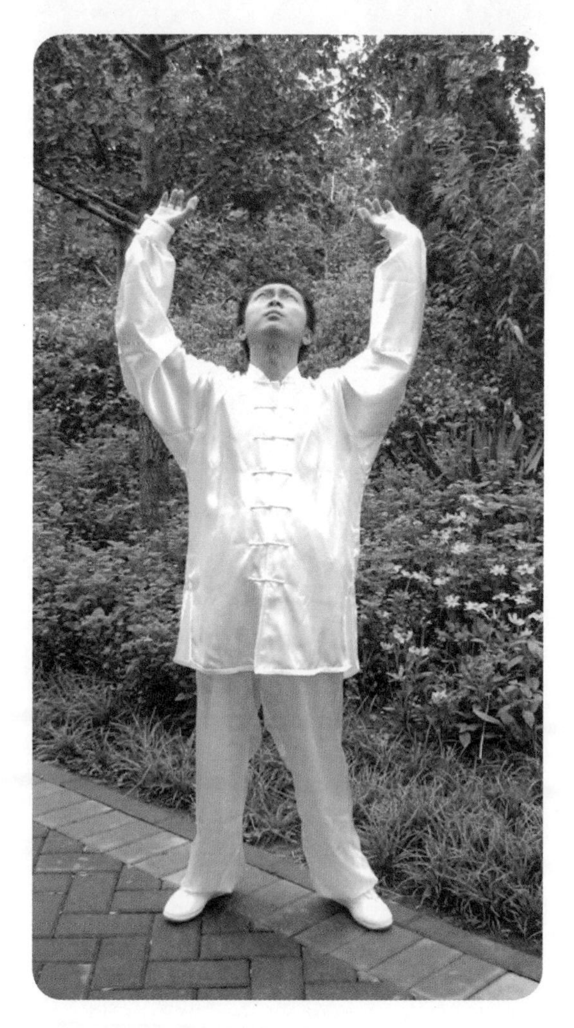

using qi gong to treat some diseases. In his famous work *On Cold Damage*, he states, "As soon as the limbs feel heavy and sluggish, use treatments such as *dǎo yǐn* (a form of qi gong), breathing exercises, acupuncture and oil massage so the nine orifices do not close up." On the foundation of qi gong and *dǎo yǐn*, his contemporary, a renowned physician named Hua Tuo (145 C.E.- 208 C.E.), created a form of exercise called *"The Five Animal Frolic"* which mimic movements of the tiger, deer, bear, ape and bird (crane). Hua Tuo told his patients to practice these exercises in order to, "free the circulation of blood and prevent disease." These five movements are still widely practiced today.

Ge Hong, a renowned physician of the Eastern Jin Dynasty (317 C.E.- 419 C.E.), thought the methods of *dǎo yǐn* should be diversified. He pointed out in his book *Bao Pu Zi's Inner Treaties* that, "Flexing or stretching, bending or looking upwards, working or lying, leaning or standing, pacing or strolling, chanting or breathing, are all methods of *dǎo yǐn*." He believed that the function of qi gong is to, "cure diseases not yet contracted and dredge discordant qi. Once it gets moving, qi will flow smoothly."

Qi gong is a practice that involves specific breathing techniques combined with movements and visualizations in order to regulate the body. These meditative exercises have been practiced in China for thousands of years and are currently practiced by millions of people around the world. They were initially created to strengthen vitality, promote longevity and prevent disease. In the last forty years, many medical facilities and research institutions throughout China have been using qi gong for rehabilitation, pain management and cancer treatment. While getting treatment for migraines, patients are advised to join a qi gong classes where they can be taught customized qi gong exercises. Various routines have been found to be effective in managing intense headaches as well as increasing energy levels[18-19]. Patients usually feel a sense of well being after practicing. Most qi gong exercises are simple and fun to learn.

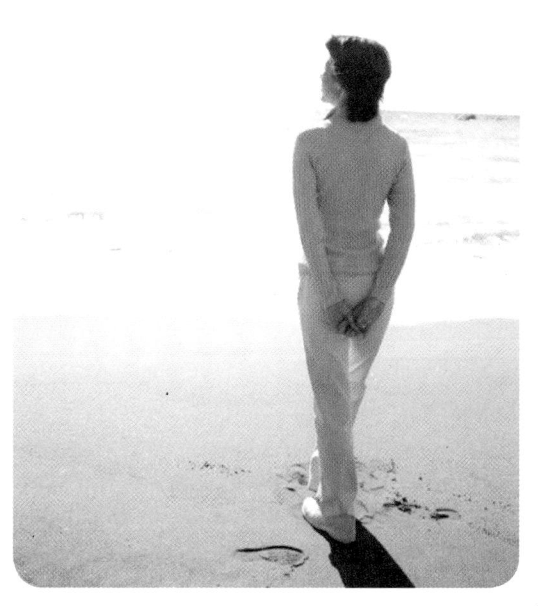

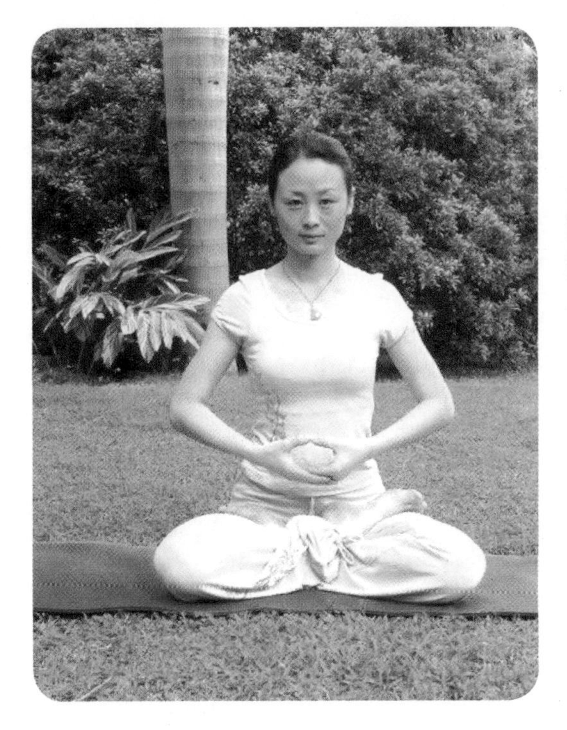

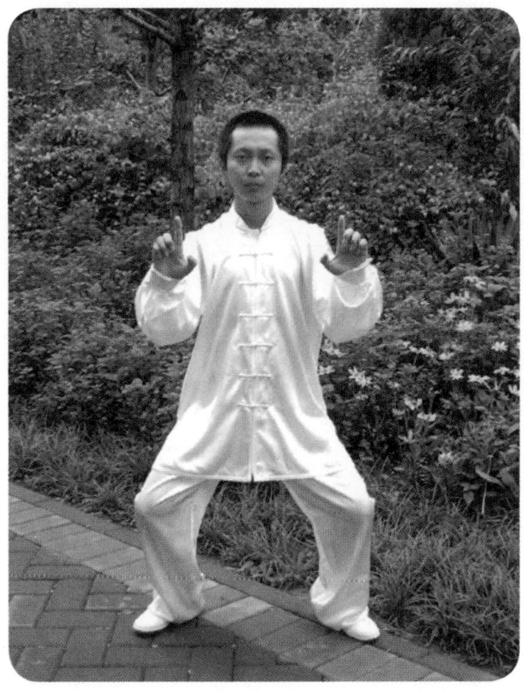

Qi gong is divided into moving and still qi gong. Moving qi gong is practiced by coordinating body movements with breath and mind. Still qi gong focuses mostly on control and coordination of breath and mind, which is more difficult for beginners. Moving qi gong, which is often mistaken for tai ji, is what most people have seen before. Qi gong is not magic, nor is it mere exercise. For centuries it has been an important element of Chinese medicine. Nearly 2,500 years ago, during the Spring and Autumn Period (770 B.C.E.- 476 B.C.E.) or the Warring States Era (475B.C.E.- 221 B.C.E.), a monograph on qi gong entitled *Inscription on Moving Qi on a Jade Pendant* appeared. This text is the first extant written reference to qi gong.

From the perspective of Chinese medical theory and practice, qi gong can supplement qi, strengthen the body, harmonize yin and yang, regulate qi and blood, smooth the flow in the channels, and calm the mind. In balancing qi, blood, yin and yang, qi gong can treat and prevent migraines.

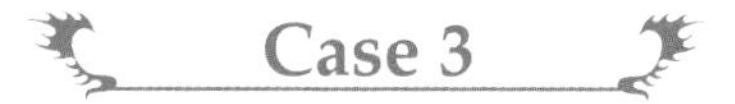

Case 3

Mr. Li is 58 years old and has had migraines for more than twenty years. His headaches were worse when fatigued. He also suffered from insomnia, dream disturbed sleep, a devitalized spirit, poor appetite, ringing in the ears, dizziness and irritability. In addition to other treatments, the doctor insisted he practice qi gong every morning. At each return visit to the clinic, his situation was better than before. After two months of taking medicine, his doctor decided that only qi gong and dietary therapy would be enough to maintain health. Presently, his migraines have stopped, his body is without disease and his spirit hearty.

The key to practicing qi gong is the regulation and coordination of body, mind, and breath. You also must choose the type suitable for your condition. In most cases you will need an instructor. Qi gong helps to stabilize the mood before a migraine attack. The following simple qi gong routines can be useful.

Internal nourishing qi gong

This qi gong routine uses a silently repeated phrase coordinated with a breathing exercise. It can regulate the nervous, circulatory and digestive systems.

Preparation

Drink some water before you start, loosen your clothes and belt. Find a relaxed posture like lying down or sitting comfortably, rid yourself of any stray thoughts and empty the mind.

Start with abdominal breathing: When inhaling, raise the tongue so it presses against the upper palate and breathe in naturally, guiding the air to the lower abdomen while visualizing it sinking down to the *dān tián*※. When exhaling, release the tongue from the hard palate so the air can leave naturally. While breathing, more attention should be paid to inhalation than exhalation. If possible, each complete breath (inhalation and exhalation) should last 30 seconds. If this is not

※ *Dān Tián* (丹田) is usually translated as "Elixir Field" but literally means "Cinnabar Field". This area, important to all forms of Asian healing, exercise, and martial arts, is located inside the abdomen, roughly 10 cm (3 in.) below the navel. This is where the root of health exists and can be nourished. There are actually three *dān tián*: this one, one in the center of the chest, and one between the eyebrows.

possible, make each breath last as long as you can and build up slowly.

Procedure

For beginners, the phrase that is recited should be short and simple, such as the Chinese phrase *"nèi yáng gōng"* (internal nourishing qi gong). First, inhale while silently reciting the first word, then hold the breath while reciting the second and third words and end with a slow exhalation. Repeat for ten minutes. To make the breaths longer and increase the benefit of the exercise, a longer phrase can be used.

Strengthening qi gong

This qi gong practice involves a breathing technique coordinated with concentration on the *dān tián*. It enriches the source qi and helps to promote good health.

Preparation

Standing is best for this routine, though sitting or lying down are acceptable. Stand with the feet shoulder-width apart, the chest slightly drawn in and the back erect, the head raised with the neck straight, the mouth slightly open, the tongue pressed lightly against the hard palate, the shoulders relaxed and the elbows at the side, both hands placed in front of the chest 15 - 20 cm (6 - 8 in.) apart as if holding a ball, the wrists slightly bent and the fingers extended.

Procedure

Regulate your breath so that it is even, and concentrate the mind on the *dān tián*. Gradually change from the normal, shallow respiration that uses the chest to deeper respiration that uses the abdomen. The breaths should become deep, gentle, even and long. After a short while, you will feel warmth and distension in the *dān tián* region. During the procedure, your mind must always be focused on the *dān tián*, and the concentration itself should be deep, aware and tension free.

The above two exercises are better practiced in the morning as this time is dominated by yang. One needs guidance to practice qi gong. If you are obsessive while practicing it may do more harm than good.

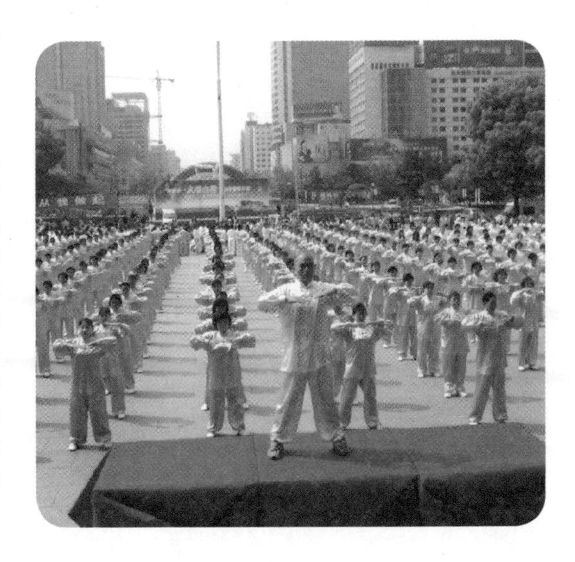

3. Translated Research

❶A group of 65 adult patients with various kinds of pain (including headaches) received qi gong therapy. The study found that qi gong was effective in relieving pain in this group of adults[14].

❷A research group conducted a literature review of the qi gong intervention studies published in English and Chinese since 1980. They were trying to determine the effectiveness of qi gong in the management of typical symptoms of pain, like painful migraines and abdominal pain. The studies selected for review showed that qi gong had a positive impact on stopping or decreasing pain both during the treatment or exercise and afterwards[20].

❸Omura et al. studied the effect inanimate objects had on different illnesses. Using muscle testing, inanimate substances were categorized either (+) or (-). Objects that were classified as (+) increased the strength of muscles and objects that were (-) weakened them. Then the effect of placing (+) objects on painful areas or muscles in spasm was compared to qi gong therapy on the areas. The results indicated that not only did the placement of properly chosen objects produce all the beneficial effects of qi gong but also enhanced the drug uptake selectively in the aea where it is necessary for the drug to be delivered for effective treatment, and reduced lead deposits in tissue[21].

❹A group of 39 adults with at least one cardiovascular risk factor (hypertension, high cholesterol, smoking habit, or diabetes) joined a tai ji quan class for one hour three times a week for twelve weeks. The purpose of this study was to determine if tai ji could improve balance, muscle strength, endurance, and flexibility. At the beginning of the study all the patients fell below the 50th percentile of fitness in their age and gender groups. Improvement in all categories was evident after six weeks and further improvement after twelve, leading to the conclusion that tai ji practice could be of great benefit to the general health of the population[23].

❺A study selected 5,159 men who were previously free of disease in order to determine the effect of physical activity on the incidence of heart disease and type II diabetes. After an average 17 - year follow-up, the authors concluded that the risk of developing either disease decreased with increasing amounts of physical activity[16]. Similar results were collected from the Finnish Diabetes Prevention Study[14] conducted in 2000.

❻Another clinical study involving 35 patients with vasomotor dysfunction in the head used qi gong directed towards acupuncture points known to be effective for headache imbalances. The effect of treatment was satisfactory to the participants in the study[22].

Other Methods of Prevention

Preventing migraines has two main benefits. The first is reducing the recurrence and severity of the headaches. This is the most important benefit. The second is to avoid drug overdose during an acute episode or side-effects during long-term use. All patients should take advantage of preventive measures, but especially those that experience more than two episodes of migraine within a month where each episode lasts more than 24 hours; cases of severe headaches; those for who drug therapy during the acute stage is not completely effective or experience a negative reaction to therapy; and where the onset of the migraine is lengthened.

Most drugs for migraine prevention include the following: calcium channel blockers, of which Flunarizine is the most potent; beta-blockers, such as Propranolol; 5 - HTA receptor antagonists, such as Pizotifen; NSAIDs, such as Indometacin, and Votalin. Chinese prepared medicines can also be used, including Correct Heaven Pill, Complex Horn Capsule, and Peaceful Brain Pill.

Preventive drug therapy needs to be employed for at least three weeks. But generally it should not surpass 9 - 12 months in order to prevent possible side-effects. If effective, another course can be

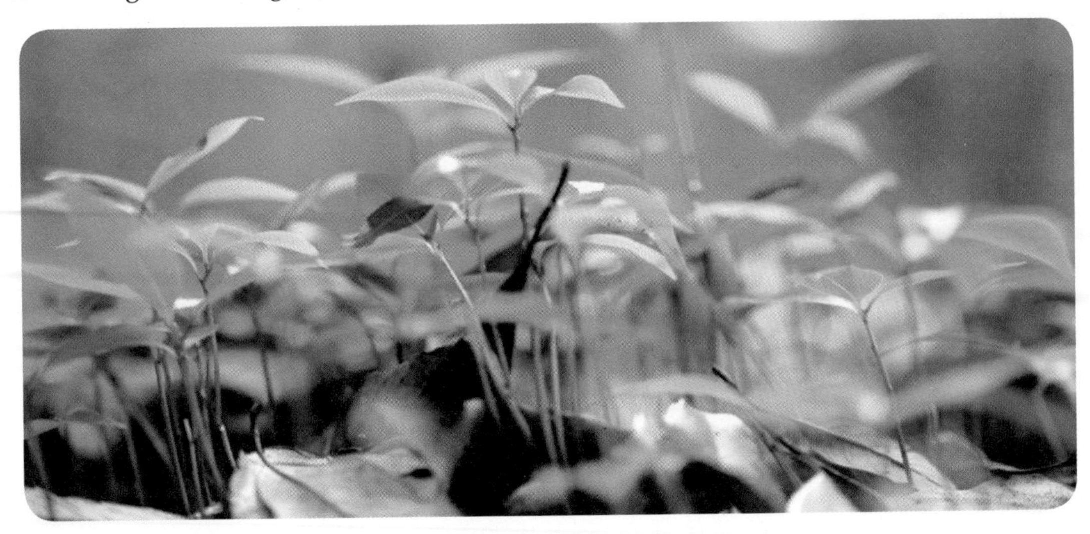

started after a break of several months. If therapy is not effective, the drug should be changed. At the same time, life-style and dietary adjustments must be made to avoid migraine triggers. With a series of comprehensive preventive therapies, many cases of migraine headache can be cured. The following suggestions cover general cautions and beneficial life-style habits that have been shown to be effective in preventing migraine headaches.

Don't combine pain-killers with cold medications

When a patient catches a cold, it is common to take an over-the-counter cold medicine. For migraine patients who take pain-killers, this can pose a serious risk. Many cold medications are a combination of numerous medicines, often including a pain-killer. If a person takes their regular pain-killer for headaches along with the pain-killer in an over-the-counter cold medication, it can lead to drug over-dose or cause the headaches to become more resilient, creating a more chronic problem.

Use caution with contraceptives

Some women get migraines when they take oral contraceptives. Some specialists believe contraceptives may increase the risk of stroke. If you have a history of migraines and stroke or heart disease in the family, and take oral contraceptives, please consult with a doctor.

Get enough vitamin B_2

Some research has found that Vitamin B_2 may reduce the duration and frequency of migraines. But the oral dose should not be more than 400 mg per day and dosage should be with the supervision of a health care practitioner. Note that the U.S. recommended daily allowance for vitamin B_2 is 1.7 mg for adult males and 1.3 mg for non-pregnant adult females.

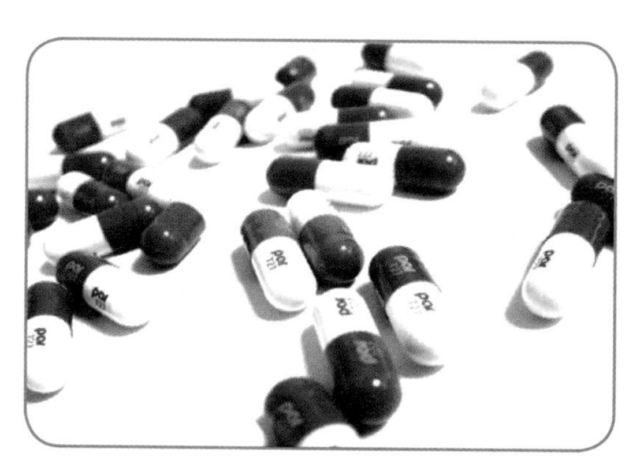

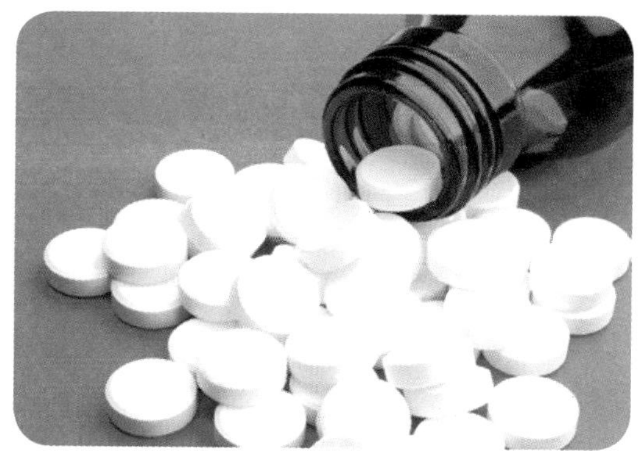

Learn to relax

If you get migraines due to work pressure and daily stress then you must take steps to relax. Warm baths, massage, and stretching, are helpful to relax muscles, as are habits such as abdominal breathing and qi gong. Learning a meditation practice can also be very helpful.

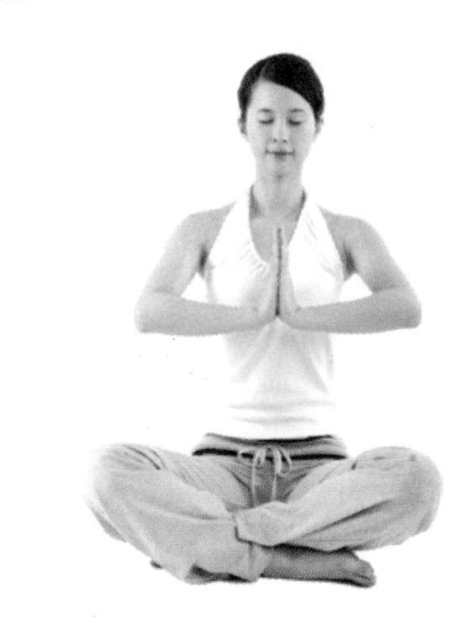

Exercise regularly

Some research has pointed out that breath training or regulated stretching (such as yoga and qi gong) can stabilize the autonomic nervous system, reducing both anxiety and muscle tension in patients with migraines.

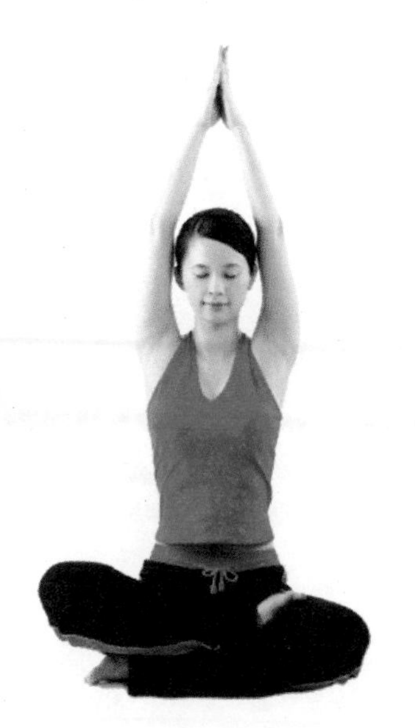

Get regular sleep

Regular sleeping habits are a must. As mentioned in earlier portions of this book and seen throughout in the case histories of real patients, lack of sleep can induce and aggravate migraine headaches.

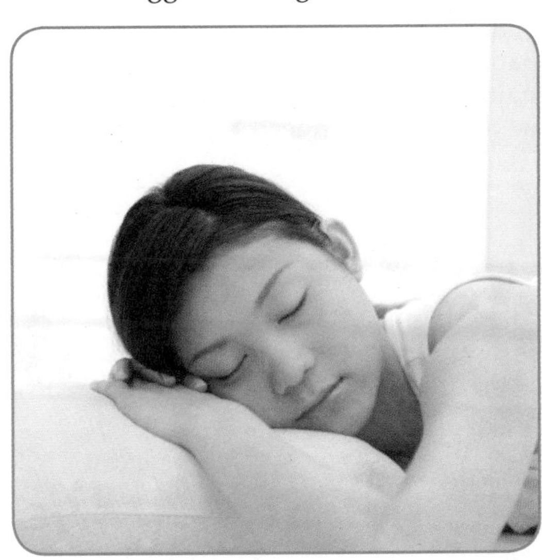

Apply heat and ice

During a migraine, one can try applying heat to the neck or ice to the forehead. The heat stimulation can help relieve muscle tension and eliminate intense pain.

Do neck and shoulder exercises

When the neck and shoulders endure tension, migraines are worse, and some people who have never had an intense headache suddenly are subjected to one. So, if you must use a computer for a long time, pay careful attention to the height of the screen and chair, and also your sitting posture. Purposely get up to stretch and relax for 10 minutes out of every hour at the computer. You may do shoulder shrugs and rotations, or other exercises learned in tai ji, qi gong or yoga.

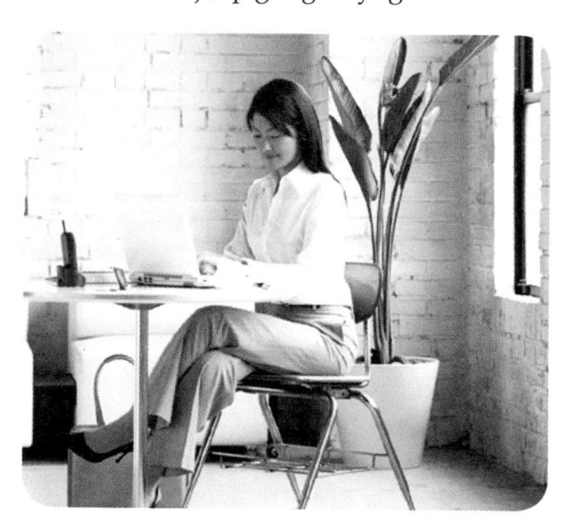

Drink water during menstruation

Severe headaches often occur just prior to or during menstruation. Women should drink more water during their period to help the body expel toxins and old blood.

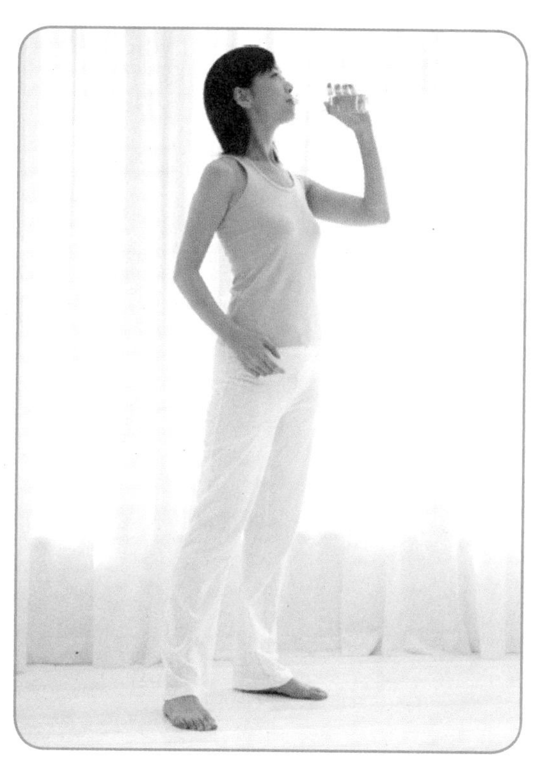

Pay attention to strong smells

Tangy or pungent smells can induce headaches. One should often open office or home windows whenever possible, and avoid places where there are strong smells, such as gas stations.

Wear sunglasses

Neurologists have determined that glare and reflected light can increase the rate of migraines by 25% - 30%. Patients should wear sunglasses to avoid UV radiation and extreme brightness.

Be quiet

Not only can intense light induce a headache, but also loud noises. Over 70% of migraine patients are sensitive to noise. That number may increase during an attack. When decorating rooms, consider sound insulation by using items such as thicker curtains that help block both light and sound.

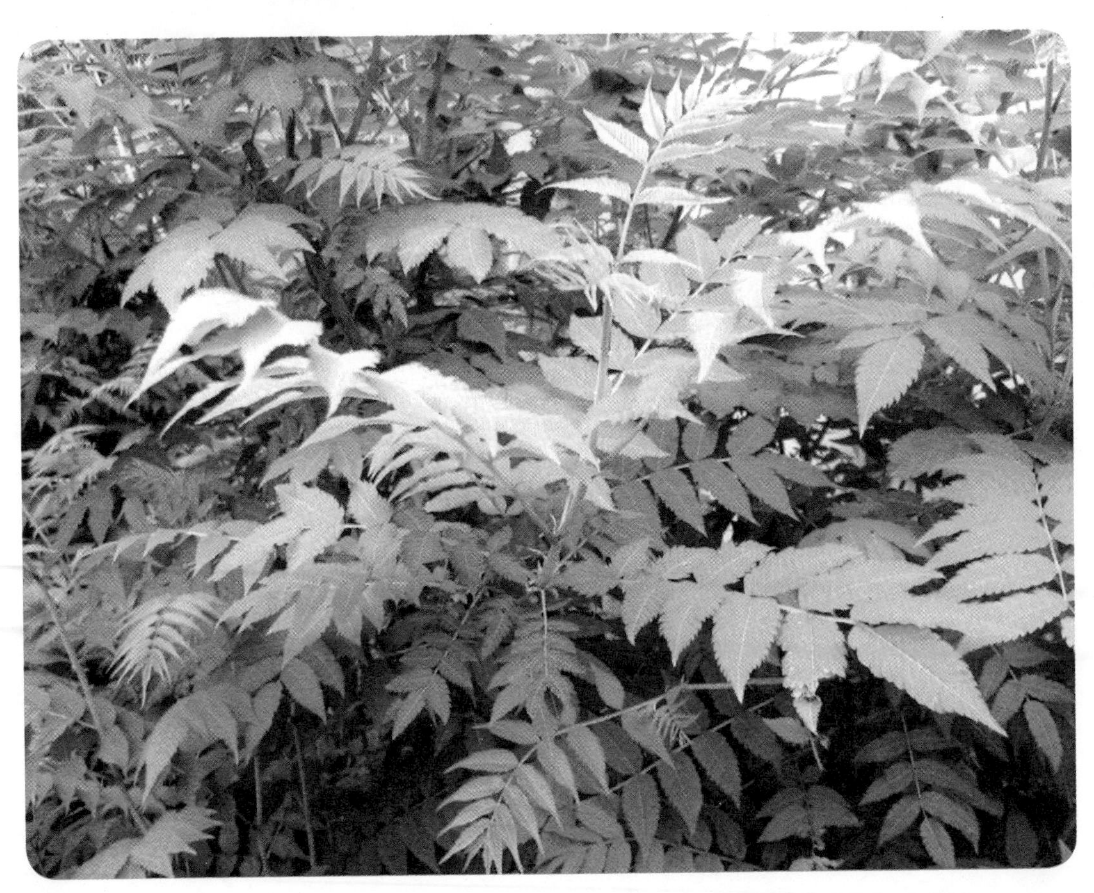

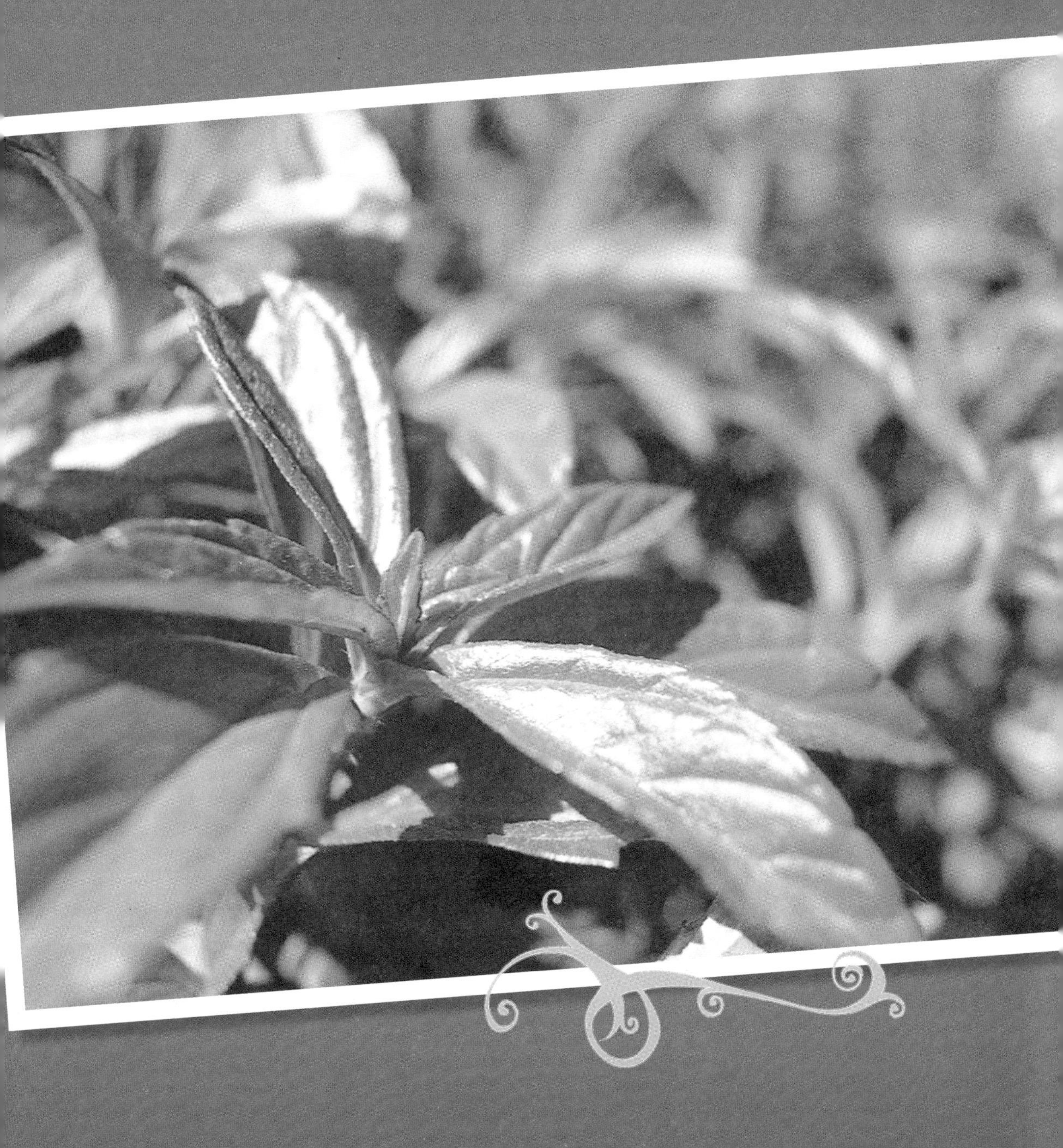

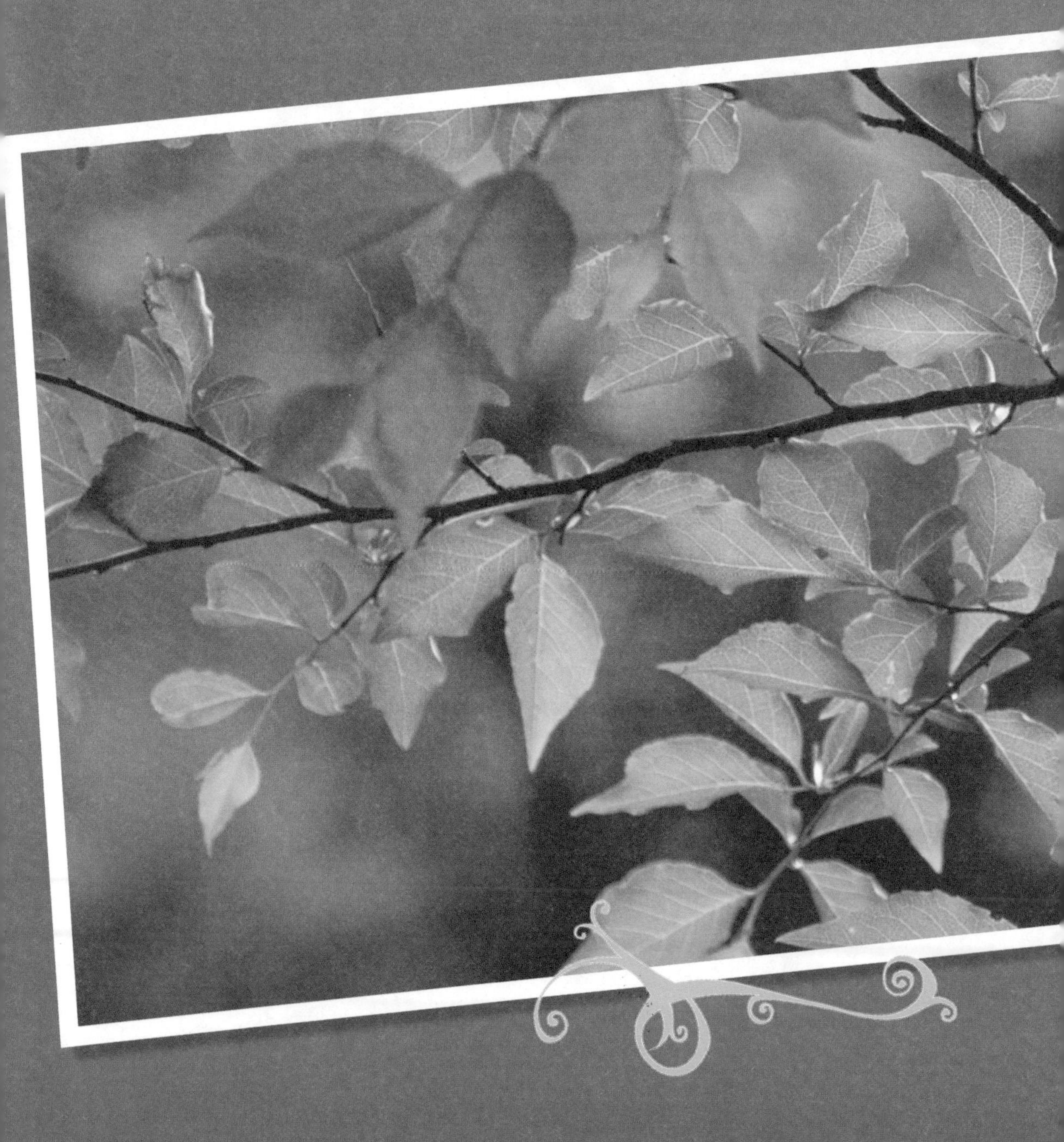

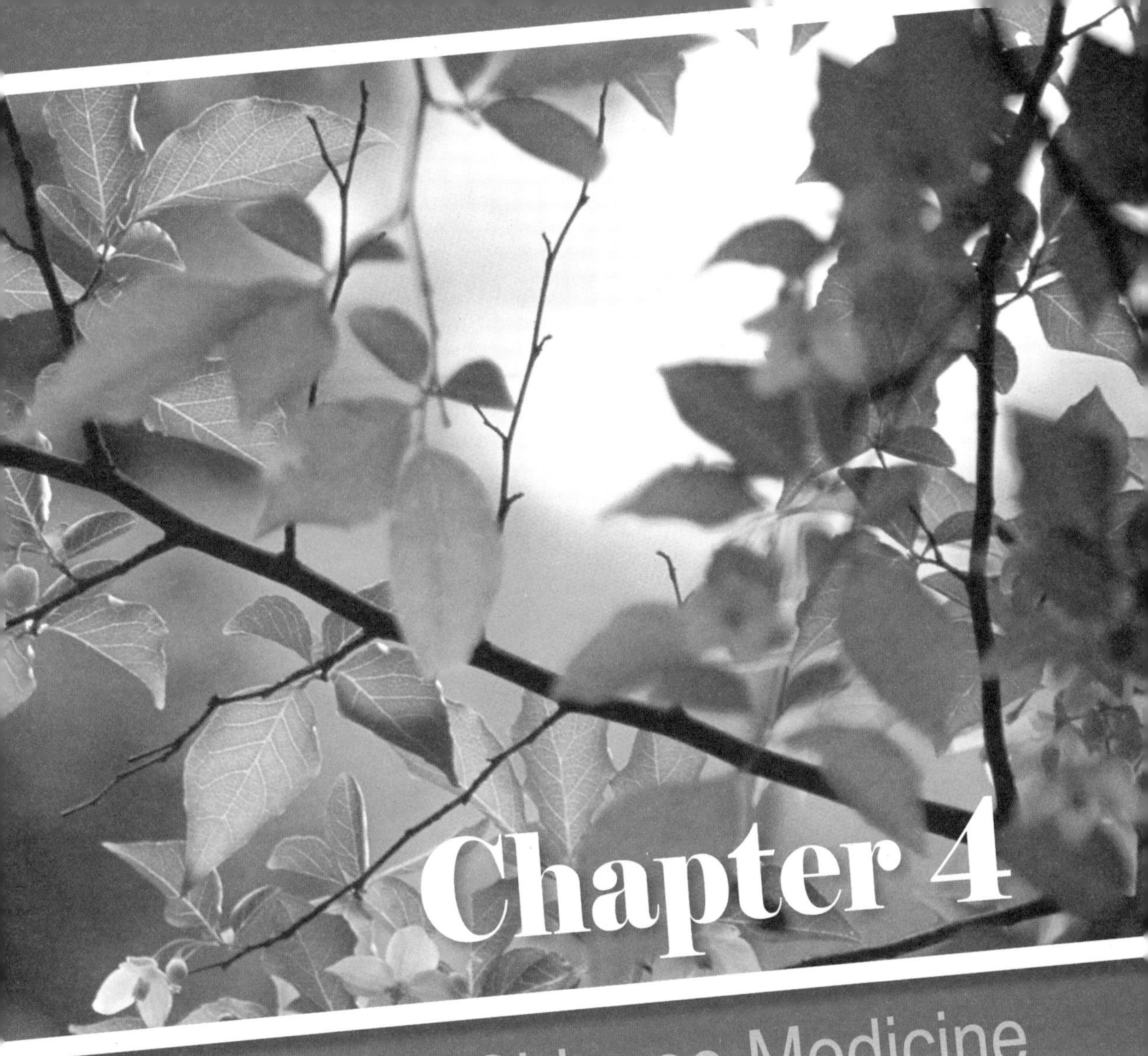

Chapter 4

How Does Chinese Medicine Treat Migraines ?

The treatment of migraine headaches is based on the pattern identified. The process of pattern differentiation is a highly intellectual, innovative, and individualized practice. Although in recent years, biomedicine has tried to achieve individualized treatment, it is fulfilled and practiced to the maximum extent in Chinese medicine. Pattern identification is why when faced with different patients with the same disease, the Chinese medical practitioner will often decide on different treatments for each case. Pattern identification can only be accomplished by using sound judgment based on an interactive, humane interview between an experienced practitioner and a patient. The ability to perform correct pattern identification is what defines a skilled doctor of Chinese medicine.

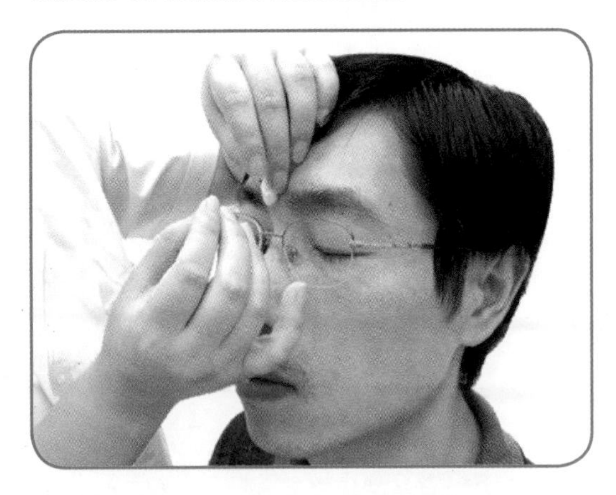

Using pattern identification, treatment methods often vary. Herbal medication is the first choice in the treatment of migraine headaches and is administered orally or sometimes applied topically. Non-herbal medication includes acupuncture, moxibustion, tui na, and other techniques. The exact treatment plan will consist of a detailed selection of herbs and an acupuncture point selection, all of which are based on the individual patient's pattern. Several treatment methods can be combined for the same patient to ensure comprehensive management.

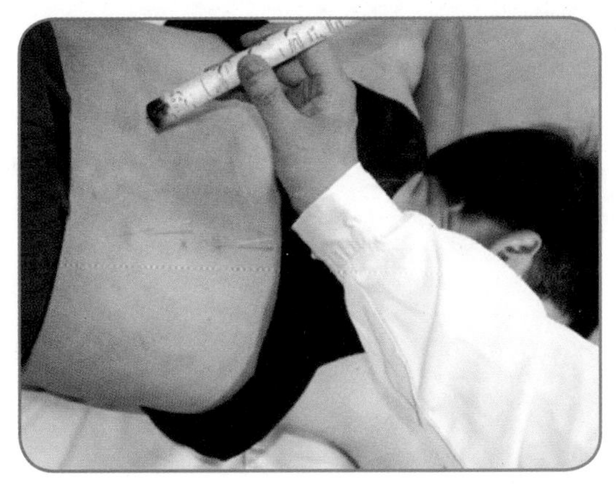

The use of modern biomedicine integrated with Chinese medicine has increased the scope of treatment available. With the help of modern technology, Chinese medicine has a better understanding of migraine headaches thanks to laboratory tests and biomedical diagnostic guidelines. Pattern identification becomes more accurate without losing its advantage of promoting the ability of human body to heal itself. Chinese medicine can provide numerous treatment methods for migraine headaches. The following sections will talk about the major ones.

Acupuncture and Moxibustion

1. What Are Acupuncture and Moxibustion?

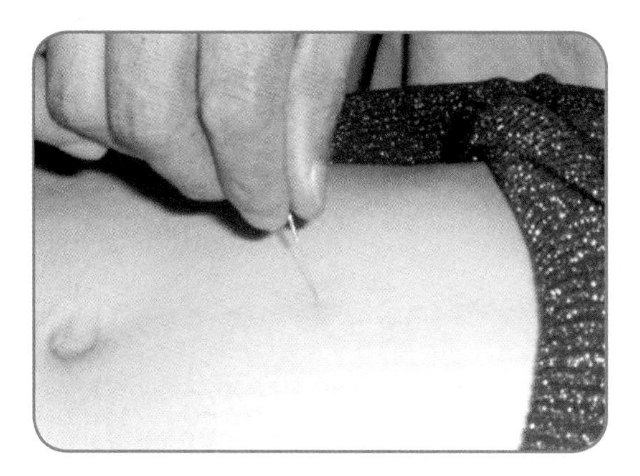

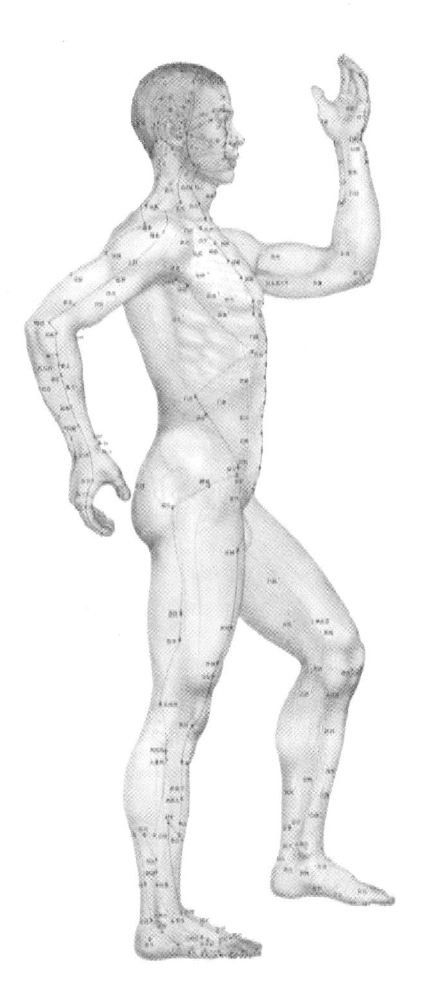

Acupuncture

Acupuncture and moxibustion are two important therapies in Chinese medicine. Acupuncture works to treat diseases by inserting fine filiform needles into places on the body surface to help the circulation of qi and blood. Acupuncture and moxibustion have been proven effective in various diseases from cardiology to psychology.

These days, acupuncture is everywhere. Searching online, one can read hundreds of reports of research involved in the scientific exploration of this ancient art. One reason these techniques are so popular is that they are absolutely safe when properly administered by a trained acupuncturist, although the thought of being needled can be unsettling to many first time patients. For most people in the West, it is difficult to understand how a fine needle inserted into the foot can relieve a headache, why a fetus's position can be reversed by needling a toe, or how puncturing a spot on the wrist can treat insomnia. All of these actions are easily explained in the language of Chinese medicine, but there are still many theories on what exactly is at work in modern scientific terms.

❶ The channels and collaterals

In the theory of Chinese medicine, the human body is an organic whole and the internal organs, external surface, and extremities are connected to each other by a network called the *jīng luò* (经络, channels and collaterals). According to this theory, the channels and collaterals connect the internal organs with the external surface and extremities by transporting qi and blood. Analogy can be made between this network and the earth's water system. With big rivers as the main thoroughfares, and the tributaries as smaller branches, the whole planet is closely connected. Acupuncture and moxibustion are applied according to this system. By stimulating the *xué wèi* (穴位, points), or the gates of this network, the human body will be influenced, moving naturally towards healing. Acupuncture points are the openings of these channels and collaterals. Inserting needles into these points will stimulate or block the flow of qi and blood and also affect the internal organs. When properly administered, the flow of qi and blood will be smoothed and organ functions will be restored. Weakness is strengthened while excess is reduced, therefore balance is restored and health regained.

Acupuncture and moxibustion are best at regulating functional disorders. In most cases the disease progression can be delayed or even stopped. If administered on a regular basis, it is also possible to reverse structural damage by promoting functional recovery. Acupuncture has been shown to be effective in clinical trials in the treatment of headache[23-26].

❷ How does acupuncture work?

The underlying mechanism behind this technique is still being researched. There exist many theories as to how acupuncture may affect the human body, and each one can explain part of the picture. In studies of its pain-relieving effect, researchers found that acupuncture blocks the impulse transmissions between the spinal cord and brain, stopping pain by closing the nerve fibers that carry impulses. This is a common theory and often referred to as the gate control theory. Various other theories also attempt to answer the question from different angles. The theory of boosting immunity states

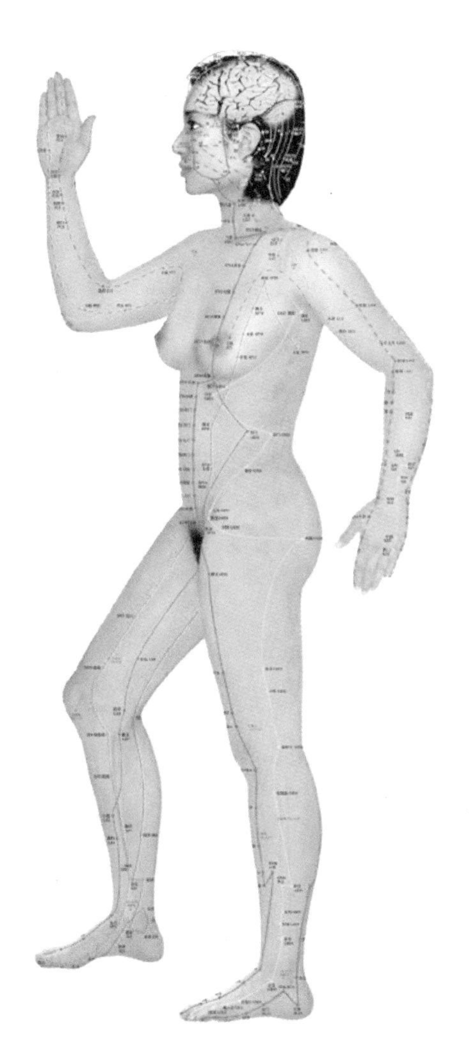

that levels of important substances such as white blood cells, antibodies, triglycerides, and gamma globulins are raised during treatment and this stimulates the immune response. Another theory states that endorphins, which act to both stop pain and promote a sense of well-being, are stimulated through acupuncture. Neurotransmitter studies show that levels of serotonin and nor-adrenaline are altered during treatment. The circulatory theory involves the release of vasodilators, which cause blood vessels to constrict and dilate.

What we can conclude from these theories is that acupuncture acts on many targets. A synthesized drug has a definite target and expected effects, together with expected side-effects as well. The function of acupuncture is done in reverse, by stimulating the body's power to regulate its own function and relieving localized symptoms. The relief of symptoms are only "side-effects" of the general changes going on at the root level.

③ Acupuncture needles

The most common acupuncture needles are called filiform needles, which are normally between 1.5 - 4.5 cm (0.5 -

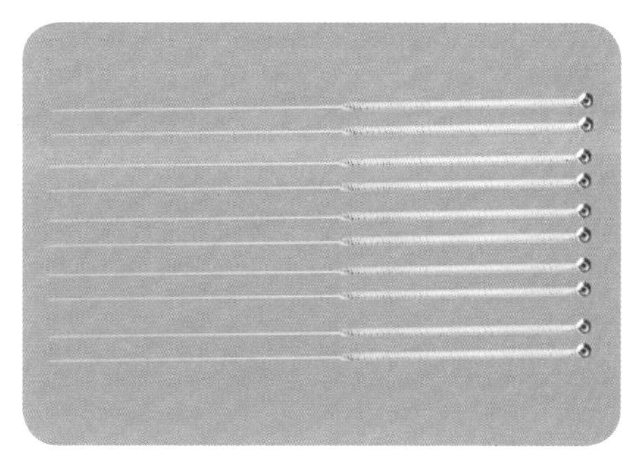

1.5 in.), but can be up to 15 cm (5 in.) depending on the location of the point to be needled and the size of the patient. The needles are usually made of stainless steel, but gold and silver needles are sometimes used. The needles are used on one patient and then disposed of in a medical waste sharps container.

④ Acupuncture positions

Different positions are used based on the points selected. As long as the patient feels comfortable, any position is suitable. Most commonly, the patient is lying on his back or stomach, though treatments are sometimes given with the patient on their side or in various sitting positions.

⑤ Clean needling practice

Acupuncturists are required to take a course called the Clean Needle Technique to train them how to handle, insert, and remove needles so both patient and practitioner are protected from any kind of contamination. The acupuncurist will wash his or her hands thoroughly with soap and water before and after treatment, and the points to be needled will be disinfected by swabbing the point with alcohol. Anything that punctures the skin will be sterile, and any other implements used in treatment will be thoroughly sanitized between patients.

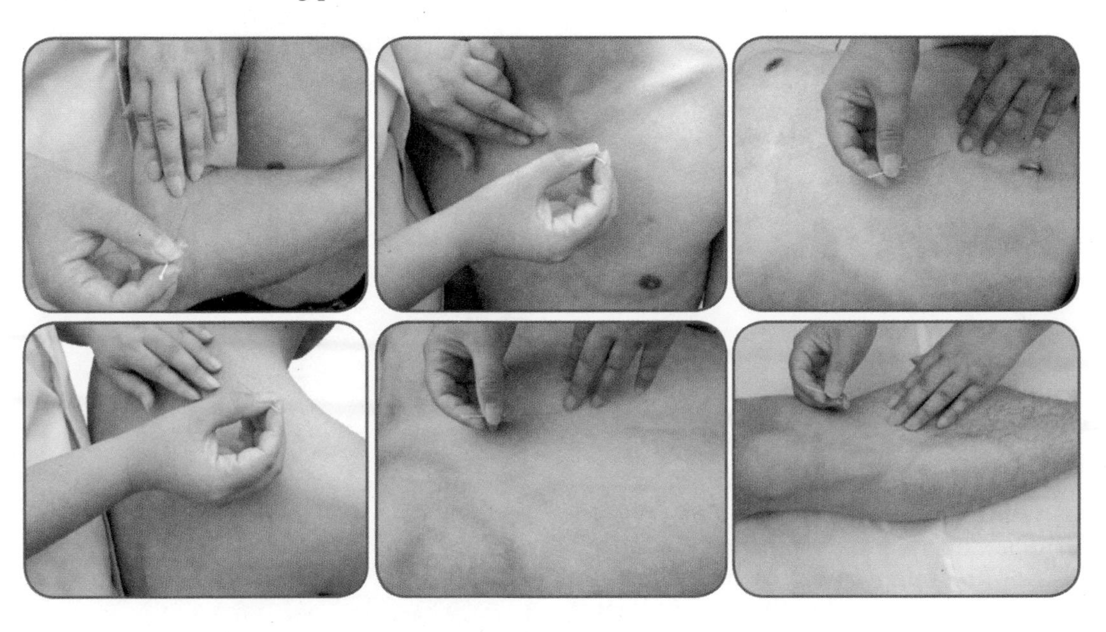

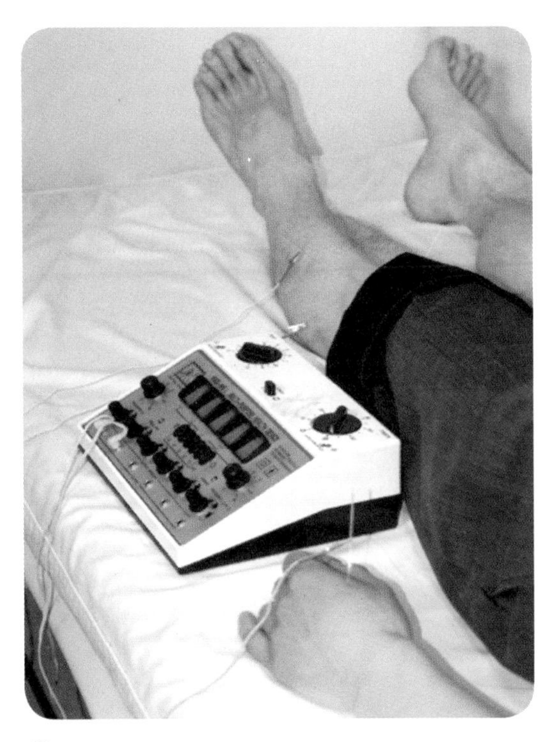

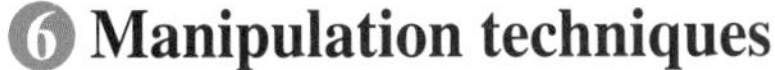

⑥ Manipulation techniques

An acupuncture treatment can be fine-tuned by using various manipulation techniques. There are several recorded methods, some vastly different in their characteristics. Some techniques pay attention to the depth the needle is inserted to. Needling shallowly has a different effect than needling deeply. Other techniques involve varying the speed or direction the needle is rotated. Fast, slow, clockwise and counter clockwise rotation techniques can all elicit different effects. Finally, many practitioners coordinate their needling with the patient's breath.

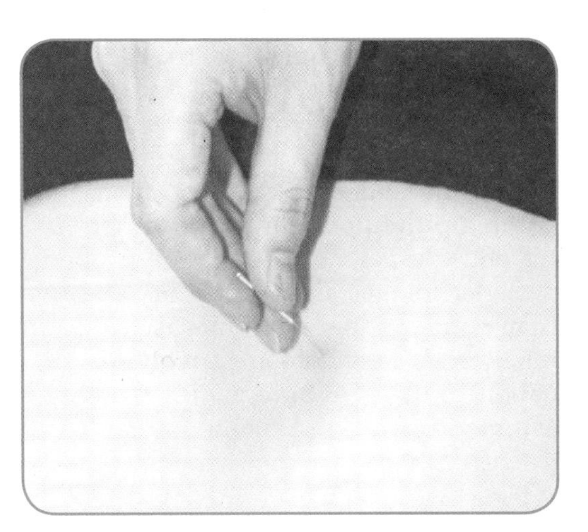

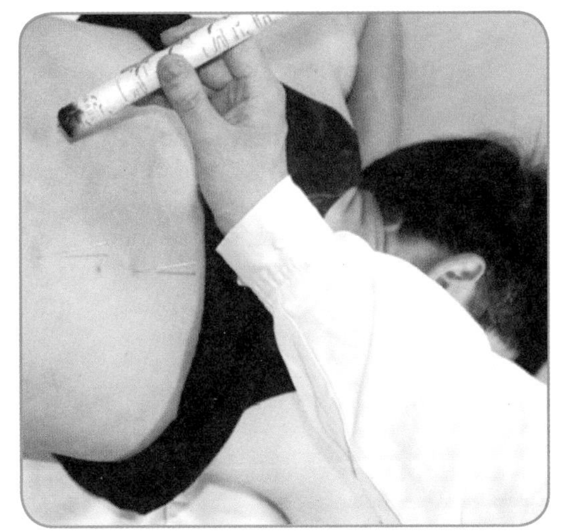

⑦ Other techniques

Though acupuncture and moxibustion are the main techniques used by practitioners of Chinese medicine, there are a variety of other techniques that may be used. These include but are not limited to cupping, *gua sha*, plum-blossom needling, and electroacupuncture. Some of these techniques may cause slight damage to the skin and tissues, but in turn, they stimulate the points much stronger and the effect lasts longer. If applied properly, these techniques are oftern more effective than conventional acupuncture for pain relief and other problems involving stagnation. In the West though, it is rare for an acupucnturist to use methods that cause extensive damage to the skin.

★ Cupping

Cupping involves the application of suctions cups to the skin either near the painful area or on a related channel. Air is vaccumed from the cups by using a burning cotton ball soaked in alcohol or by using modern cups that use manual air suction. There is no pain involved in cupping, although the sensation of suction is sometimes strange the first time.

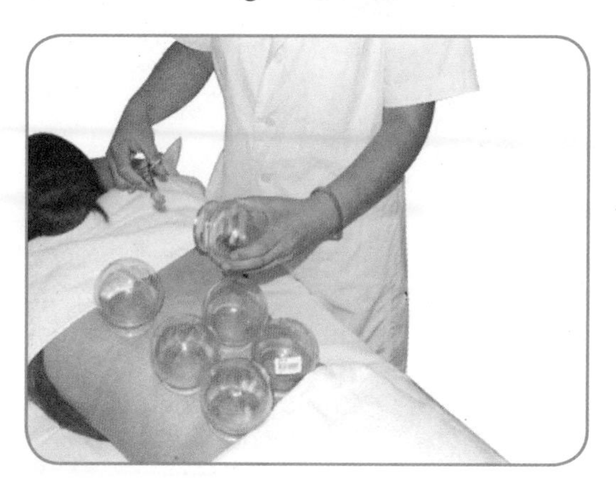

★ Plum blossom needle

The dermal needle is also known as the "plum-blossom" or "seven-star" needle. It is made of 5 to 7 stainless steel needles arranged in a pattern like the seed pod of the lotus flower, and fixed on one end of a plastic handle. The dermal needle is tapped on the skin to stimulate circulation and promote qi movement in the channels. These needles are usually either entirely disposable or come with a reusable handle and disposable tips.

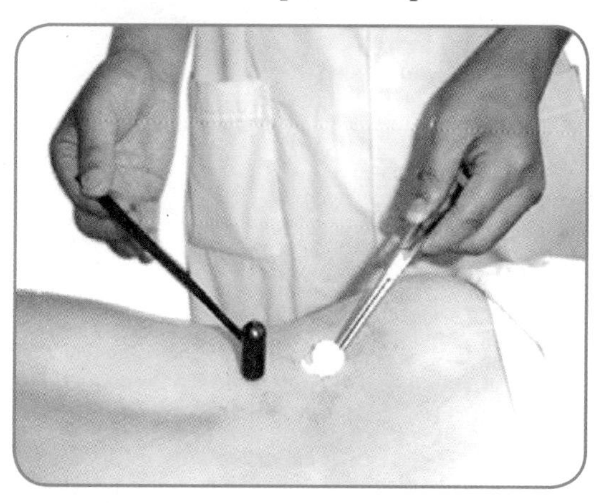

★ *Gua sha*

Gua sha is a technique of rubbing the skin and is used in many cultures. It is usually used for pain that is recent and hasn't had time to move deep into the body. The rapid, light scraping techniques are not painful, but will elicit slight red-

ness or bruising in the area. These bruises are very superficial, not painful, and are a sign that the congestion causing pain has been activated and is leaving the body.

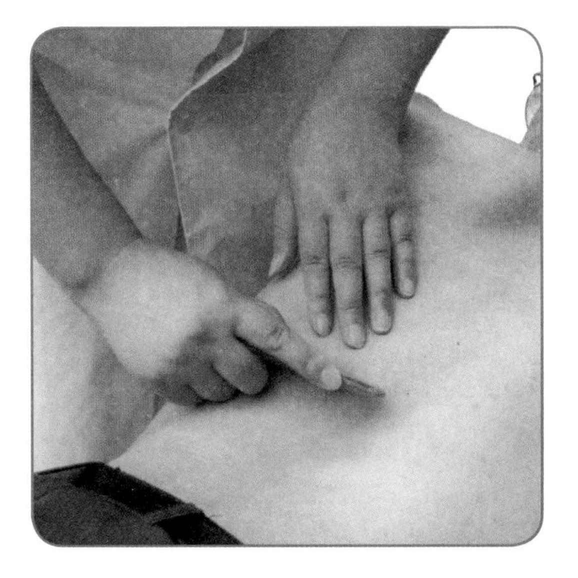

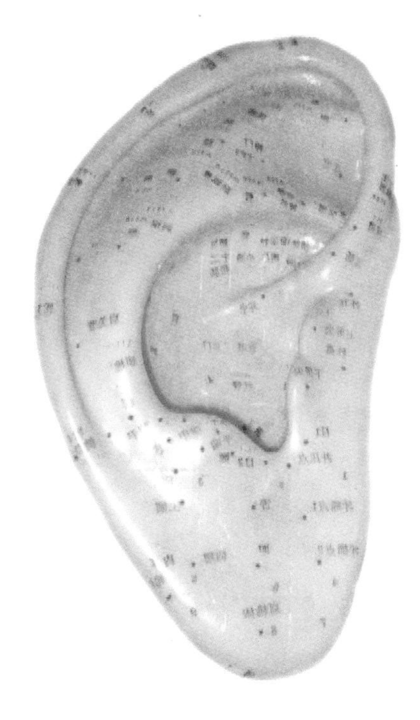

★ **Scalp acupuncture**

Scalp acupuncture is a therapy in which specific areas on the scalp are needled to prevent or treat diseases. Scalp acupuncture does not follow the traditional mapping of acupuncture points, but relies on more recent evaluation of the neurological functions in the brain. It may be used for conditions such as stroke or paralysis, as well as migraine.

★ **Ear acupuncture**

Ear acupuncture is a new addition to Chinese medicine's treatment arsenal. Similar to reflexology, the ear represents a micro-system of the entire body. The points on the ear are mapped out as if the ear was a curled up human figure upside down, with the head as the lobe and the legs curled up to form the top of the ear. Although there are specialists who mainly use ear acupuncture, most practitioners use it as a helpful adjunct therapy. A popular technique is to place a small seed, metal pellet, or tiny needle on an ear point and keep it in place with a small piece of tape. These objects will then provide a constant stimulation to the points chosen. This convenient form of therapy allows for around the clock treatment. Normally the tape is taken off in three or four days.

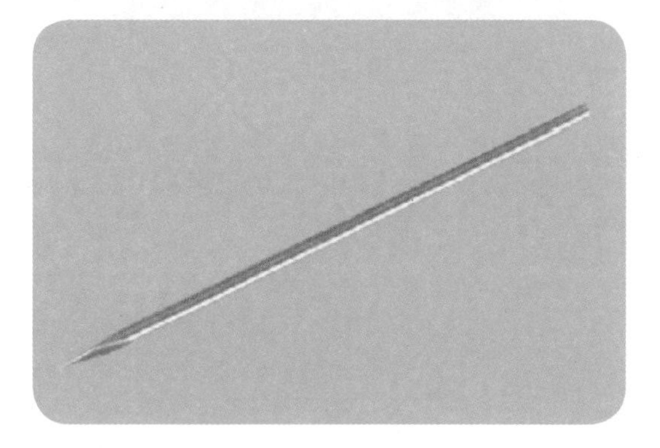

★ Three edged needle

The three edged needle is a needle with a thick, round handle, triangular body, and sharp tip, and is used for pricking a point to cause slight bleeding. Usually only a few drops of blood are let out to help release stagnant blood or heat. Strict safety measures are taken to prevent accident or injury.

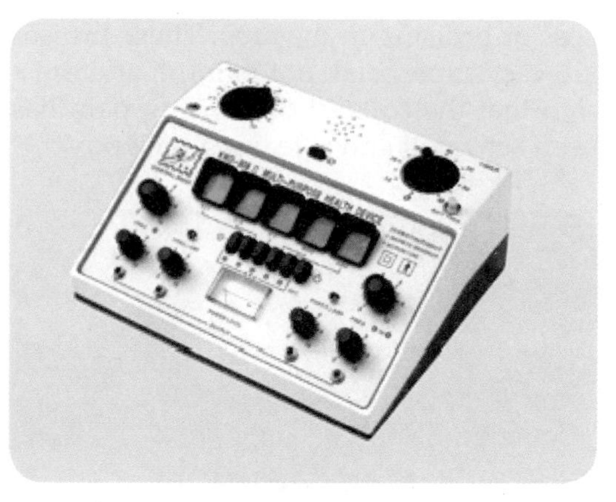

★ Electroacupuncture

Electroacupuncture has become commonly used in recent years. Practitioners use an apparatus that allows an electrical impulse to be sent through the needles to mimic constant manipulation. Practitioners are trained to operate the machines safely and the amount of power sent through the needles is very small. Electroacupuncture is commonly used for problems that require constant needle stimulation. The machine will allow the practitioner to do other work while the point is receiving stimulation.

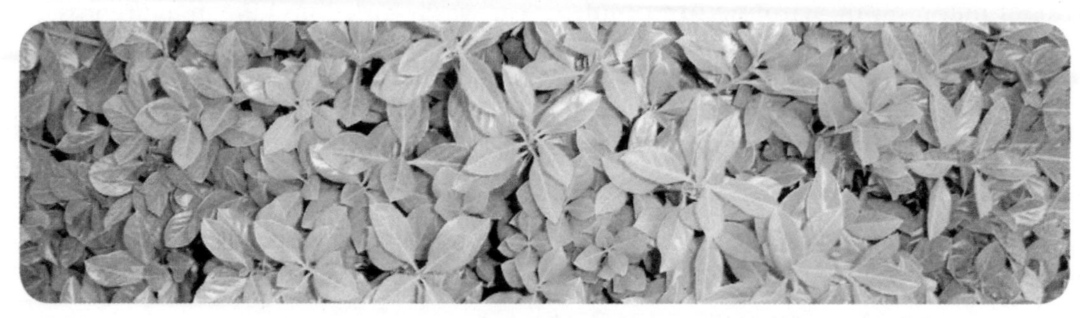

8 Commonly used points

There are hundreds of points on the human body, most of which are situated along fourteen main channels. Some of the points are more commonly used than others. The points selected in the treatment of migraines can vary greatly, according to the patterns, the patient, and the practitioner's training. The final point selection depends on your specific condition and the practitioner's judgment.

The action of every point is to regulate yin and yang, the difference is in what exact way each point works. Some points work on the qi aspect, while others may work on the blood; some are warming, and others are cooling. Most point functions have not been verified by modern research, but for some of the more important points, some research has been done. For example, LI 4 (*hé gŭ*) is a point commonly used in clinic. It is effective in the treatment of treating pain as it has an effect on the circulation of qi and blood. Puncturing this point can regulate qi and blood to stop pain. Modern research has found that using this point has a powerful impact on brain chemistry as well as a variety of neurologic functions. One of the reasons for the effectiveness of acupuncture therapy on pain is its impact on brain chemistry[27].

Below are some photos and descriptions of commonly used points in the treatment of migraine headaches. Of course all patients are different, so not everyone will get all of these points. But since some of these are major points, everyone is likely to experience at least a couple of these points during the course of treatment. According to pattern differentiation and diagnosis, migraines can be divided into the six patterns listed in chapter two. These include headache due to wind, deficiency, blood stasis, and dampness.

风池 ***Fēng Chí* (Gallbladder 20)**

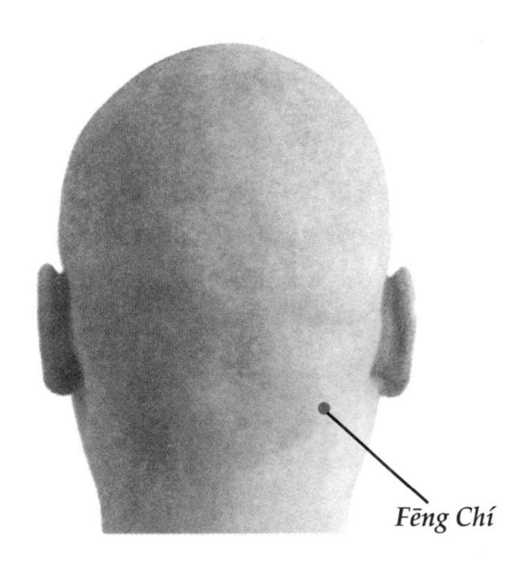

GB 20 (*fēng chí*), which means "Wind Pool", is one of the most important points on the gallbladder channel and very useful in treating headaches. It is most often used in migraines due to wind, rising liver-yang, or those that affect the back of the head. Stimulating the point can also treat a variety of disorders involving the neck and head such as dizziness, eye diseases, problems with the cervical vertebrae, and ringing in the ears.

GB 20 (*fēng chí*) is located in a depression behind the ear, just under the skull, and between the two major muscles of the side and back of the neck.

太阳 ***Tài Yáng* (Extra Head-Neck 5)**

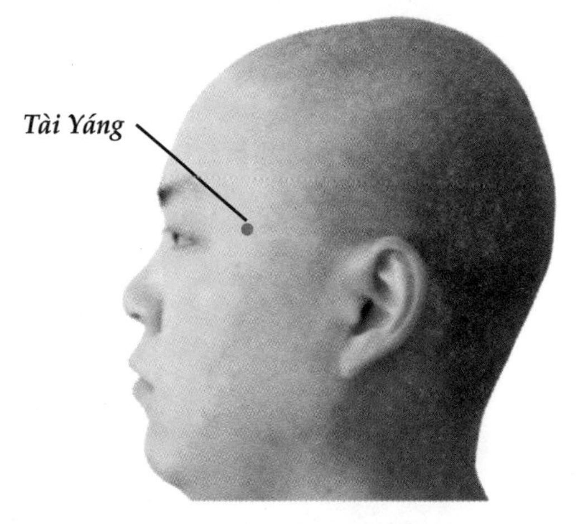

Tài yáng is the word for the sun in Chinese, but literally means "Ultimate Yang". It is considered an "extra point" because it does not lie on one of the main fourteen channels. Famous Shaolin martial artists say that if *tài yáng* is hit correctly and with enough force, a person will lose consciousness or even die. Modern medical research results have proved that hitting *tài yáng* can indeed have this effect. As an acupuncture point, it is effective in treating diseases due to excess yang in the head such as headache, tiredness of the eyes and also toothache. *Tài yáng* is absolutely necessary in the treatment of migraines.

Tài yáng is located in front of and slightly above the ear, on the temple, in the noticeable depression about one inch lateral from the eye.

鱼腰 ***Yú Yāo* (Extra Head-Neck 4)**

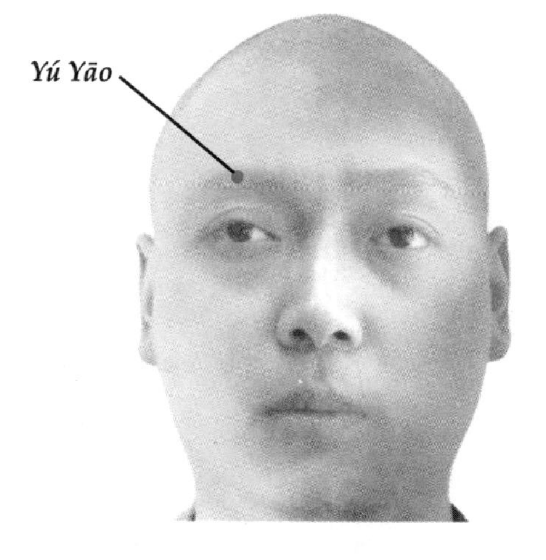

Yú yāo is also an extra point. Its name has the odd meaning of "Fish Waist". The point is located on the mid-point of the eyebrow, and the ancient Chinese saw a similarity between the curve of the eyebrow and the soft curve of a belly of a fish. *Yú yāo* would then be located in the middle of that fish, about at it's waist. In clinical practice the point treats many facial disorders such as conjunctivitis with swelling and pain, drooping eyelid, facial palsy and trigeminal neuralgia as well as headaches.

The accurate location of *Yú yāo* is above the pupil, in the middle of eyebrow.

The following are acupuncture points that are located on parts of the body away from the head that can be used to treat migraine headaches:

合谷 ***Hé Gǔ*** **(Large Intestine 4)**

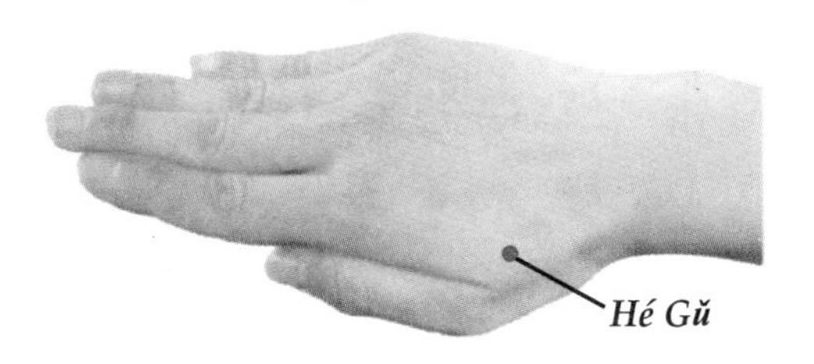

This point is often used because of its ability to stop pain and improve the circulation in the channels. It is one of the main acupuncture points used for anesthesia when head and neck surgery is performed. *Hé gǔ* is frequently used for headaches, but also is often selected in cases of eye redness or soreness or pain, swelling and pain of the throat, toochache, deafness, painful menstruation, abdominal pain and arm pain.

Hé gǔ is located on the hand, in the muscle between the thumb and forefinger. When needled, a strong sensation is often felt that can extend to the elbow, shoulder and even the face.

太冲 ***Tài Chōng*** **(Liver 3)**

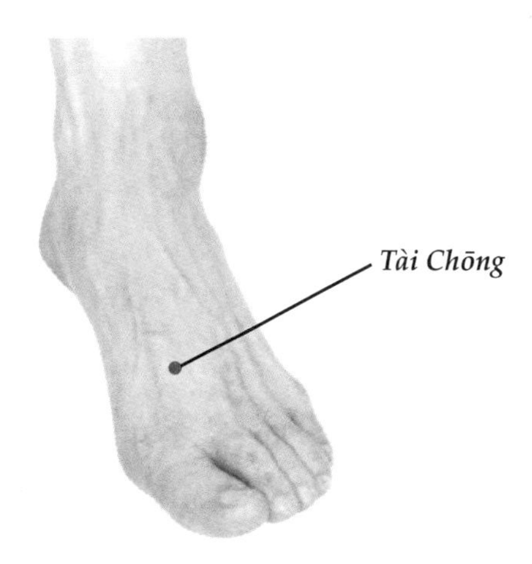

The indications for this point include headache, dizziness, insomnia, eye-redness and swelling, and swelling and pain of chest and ribs. It can clear away heat from the liver channel, and is especially effective for pain related to excessive rising of liver yang.

It is located on the foot in the depression between the bones of the big toe and the second toe.

太溪 ***Tài Xī*** **(Kidney 3)**

On the kidney channel, this point is used in cases where the kidney is deficient. These patients often experience the following symptoms along with their headaches: a dry and sore throat, toothache, ringing in the ears, insomnia, nocturnal emission, impotence, irregular menses, and soreness of the lower back and knees.

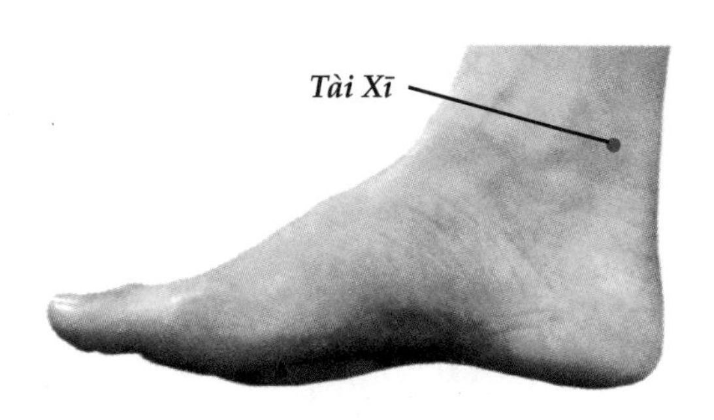

It is located between the inner ankle bone and the Achilles tendon. Moxibusiton is often used on this point.

Moxibustion

Moxibustion is the application of heat using a small bundle of tightly bound herbs which are then burnt over targeted acupuncture points. In Chinese medicine, the purpose is to stimulate a point, and is not only accomplished by using an acupuncture needle. Therefore several methods can be used such as heat, massage, as well as modern methods that use laser, light and electricity. By applying heat stimulation to certain points, the practitioner can regulate the yin-yang balance of the internal organs to prevent disease, heal the body, and preserve health. Based on the same theories as acupuncture, moxibustion is a useful treatment method.

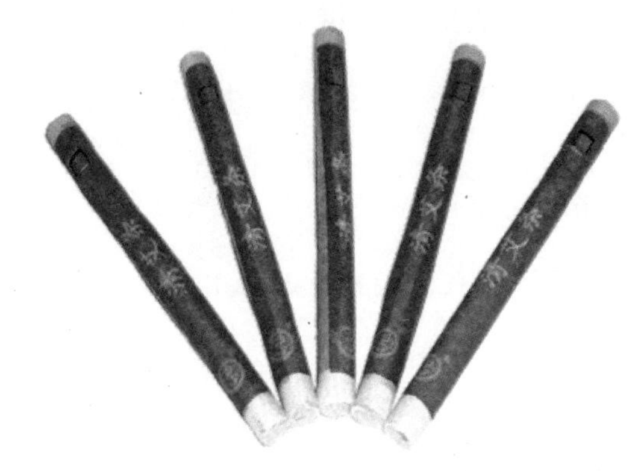

The material used in moxibustion is usually made of Artemisia leaves, commonly called mugwort. The Chinese herbal medical classic *Miscellaneous Records of Famous Physicians* states that Artemisia leaves are bitter, slightly warm, without any toxicity, and should be used in moxibustion to treat all types of diseases. Artemisia leaves, being warm in nature, can promote the flow of qi and blood, remove dampness and cold, and dissolve masses and accumulations in order to cure illness, prevent disease and maintain health. Moxibustion has been used for thousands of years, longer even than stone needles, the ancient precursors to modern acupuncture needles. Like acupuncture, much research has been done on the therapeutic effects of moxibustion and it is widely used as an effective supplement to acupuncture treatment. The leaf is also taken internally as tea, most often for bleeding and menstrual disorders.

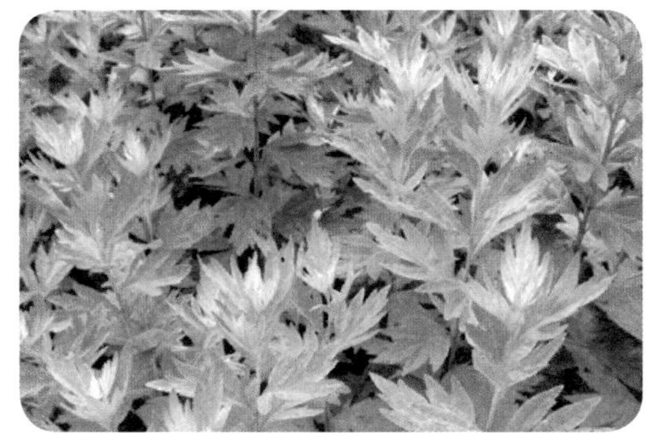

Mugwort Leaves

In the language of Chinese medicine, moxibustion can regulate yin and yang by supplementing yang, supplementing qi and blood, improving circulation in the channels, helping the body fight invading pathogens, and regulating the internal organs. These functions illustrate how moxibustion can prevent disease and delay aging.

1 Different types of moxibustion

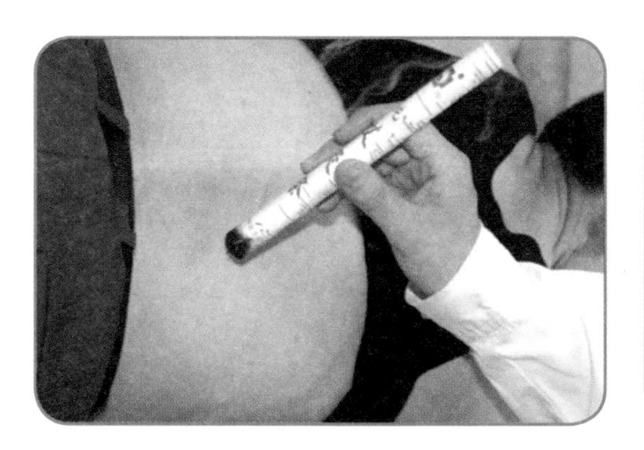

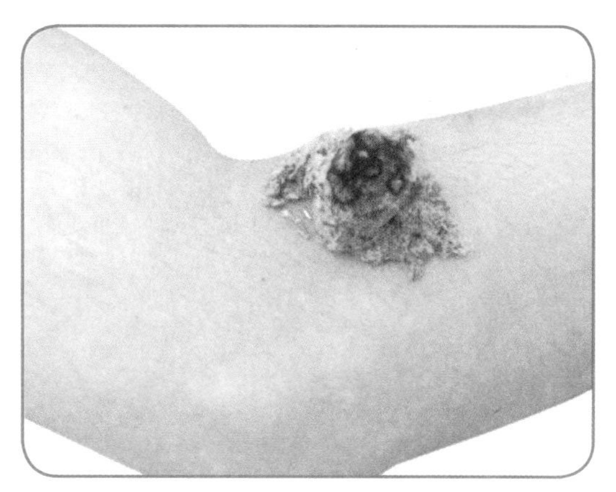

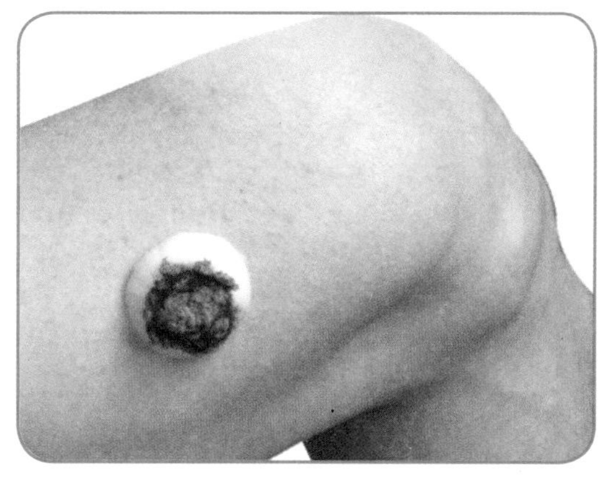

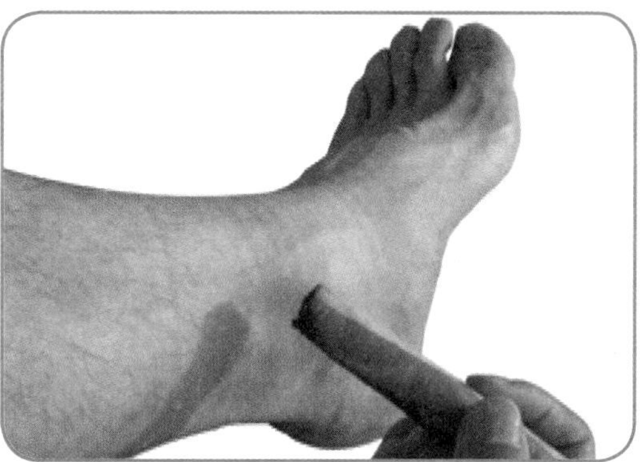

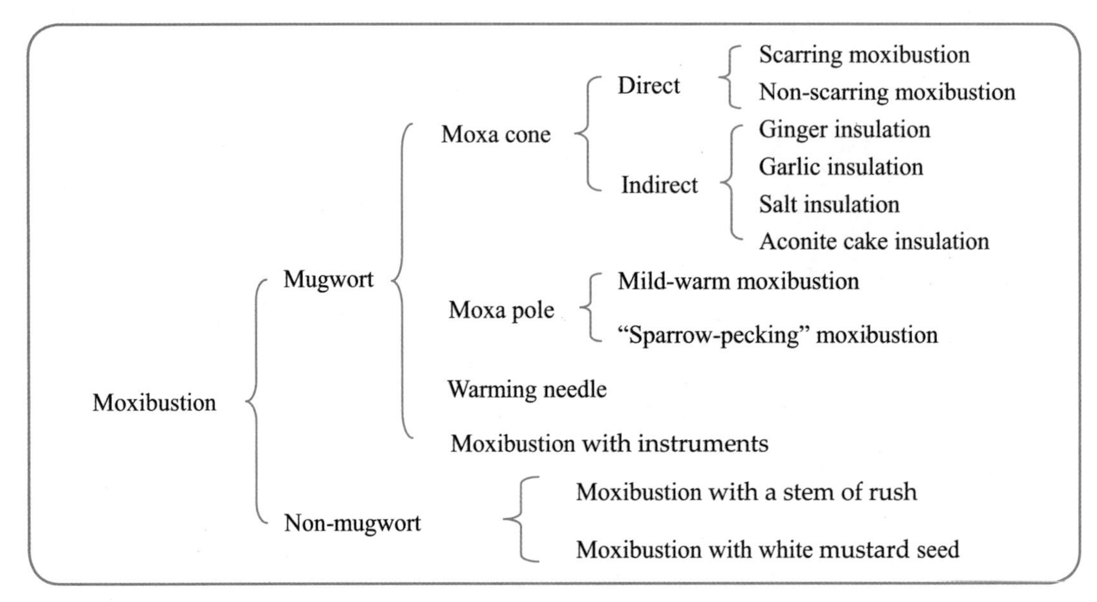

The two main types of moxibustion are direct and indirect.

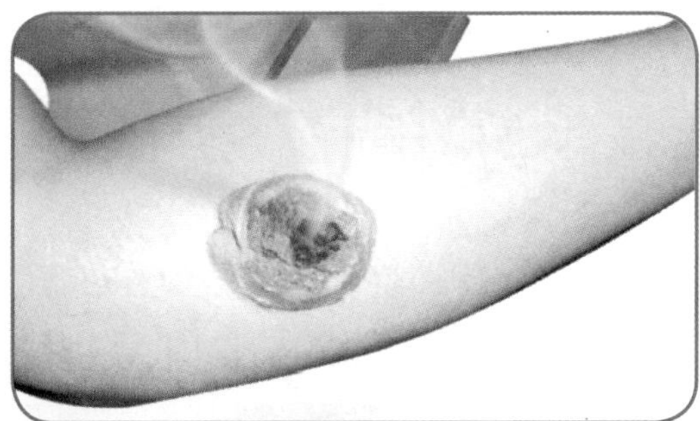

★ Indirect moxibustion

The most common form of heat therapy is indirect moxibustion. It involves either the use of a cigar-shaped moxa pole, or the burning of moxa cones on top of a layer of ginger, garlic, or salt. With a moxa pole, a practitioner holds the stick roughly 4.5 cm (1.5 in.) above the skin and holds it in place until the skin becomes red or appears congested. When garlic, ginger, or salt is used with moxibustion, they provide a buffer from the heat of the moxa as well as adding their own properties to the therapeutic effect. These forms of treatment do not usually cause severe pain or leave any blisters or scars, though the skin

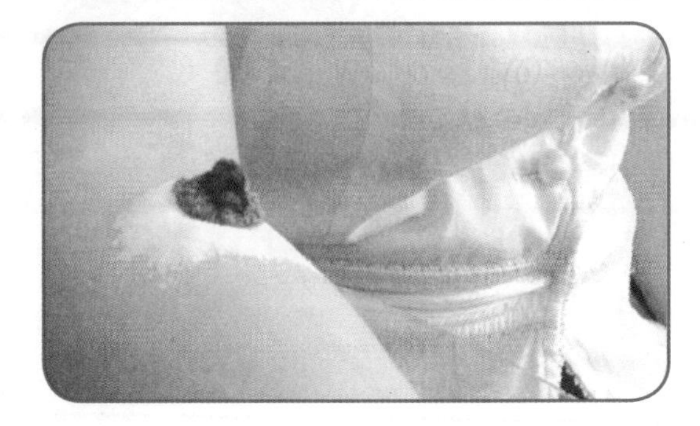

may remain red for a while, which is considered a desirable side-effect.

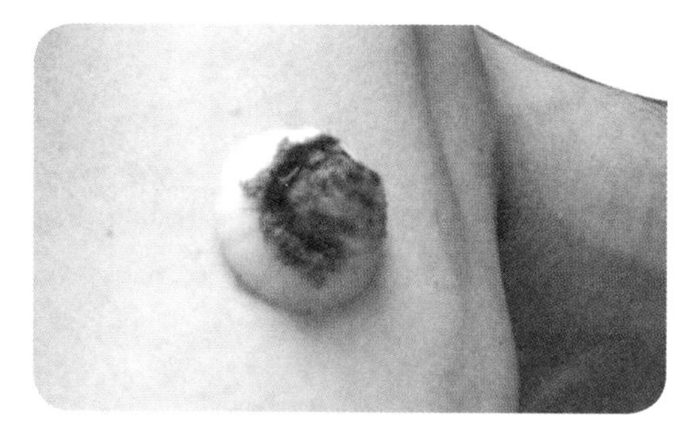

★ **Direct moxibustion**

Direct moxibustion uses moxa cones. These are usually shaped to roughly 1.5 cm (0.5 in.) high, placed directly on acupuncture points, Lit, and left in place until the cone is extinguished or until the area becomes hot. This is a strong form of treatment and can produce pain, blisters, and even scarring. Some Chinese and Japanese traditions still deliberately induce scarring, which is believed to have the strongest effect. This form of treatment is usually reserved for very serious cases being treated by experienced practitioners.

★ **Moxibustion with yangsui brush**

Recently in the clinic, moxibustion with yangsui brush is being used to treat various kinds of diseases. Various medicinals are mixed together with refined moxa and licorice extract, and then compressed into a sliver-like brush. Treatment using the yangsui brush is faster than conventional moxibustion, and also produces less smoke and fumes. Treatment only takes a couple of minutes compared with over fiteen minutes with a moxa pole or cone. Often special medical paper is used together with the yangsui bursh in order to protect the skin and strengthen the medicinal action.

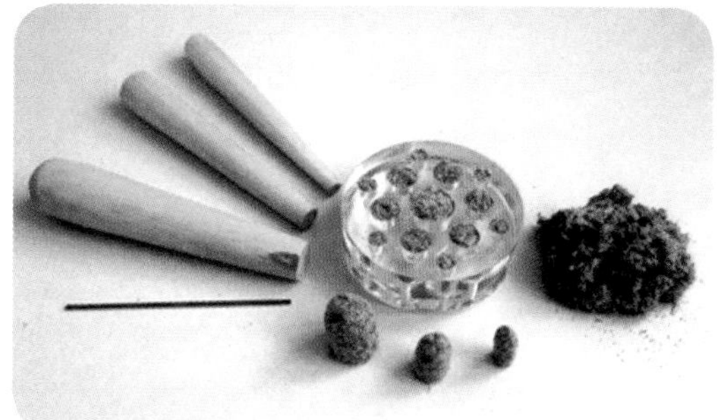

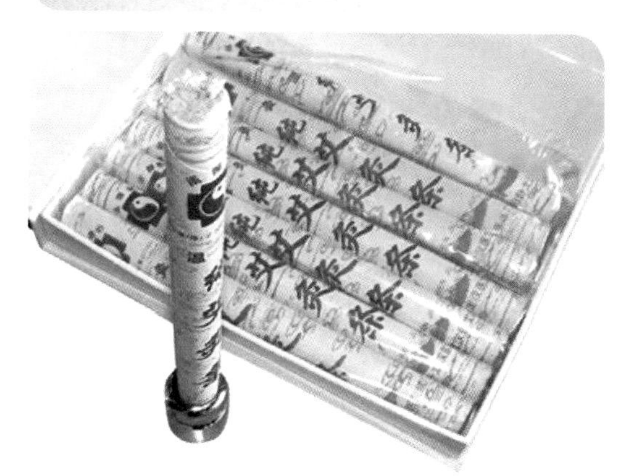

Practitioners may also place a moxa cone on top of an acupuncture needle and burn it in a process called "warming needle". This takes the heat directly into an acupuncture needle where it can disperse in the tissue several centimeters deep. If good ventilation is not available, heat can also be applied to points from an electrical source designed specifically for this. For people who have asthma or other respiratory problems, smokeless moxa can be used.

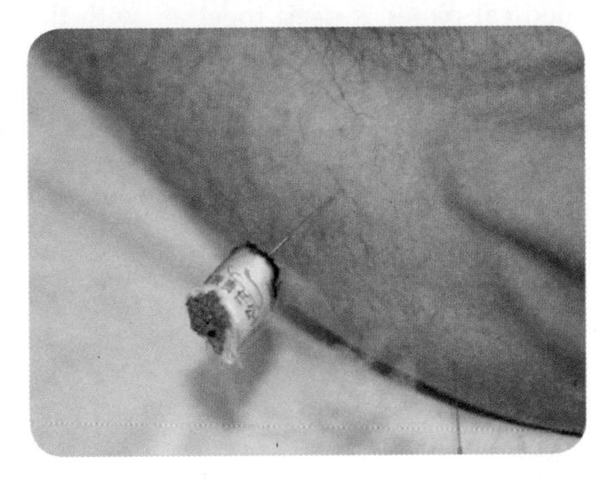

Moxibustion is not for everyone. It is indicated mainly for patients suffering from cold or stagnation. It is not used on patients diagnosed with excess heat. Since patients with migraine headaches often present with blood stagnation patterns, moxa is very useful and often used. It can also help relax muscle tension.

2 Precautions for treatment

All acupuncturists today are trained in safety issues regarding their patients. The following are some general rules the patient should be aware of. Patients should also feel free to ask questions regarding safety issues they are concerned about as they arise during treatment or consultation.

- Patients who are very hungry, fatigued or nervous should not receive treatment. For patients who are weak, strong stimulation is not allowed.

- It is not suitable to needle points on the abdomen or lower-back of pregnant women. Certain points are also specifically forbidden to use during pregnancy.

- Points on the vertex of infants should not be needled when the fontanels are not closed.

- Extra precaution must be taken for any patient who has bleeding disorders.

- Areas of infection, ulceration, scars or tumors on the skin will not be needled.

- When needling more fragile areas such as points near the eyes, neck, chest, back and ribs, great care must be taken to not injure the tissue or organs.

2. What Will Treatment Be Like?

After collecting detailed information about a patient's symptoms, signs, lifestyle and living and work environment, as well as looking at the tongue and inspecting the pulse, the Chinese medical practitioner will identify the pattern of disharmonies present. Based on this pattern identification, an optimal treatment protocol will be drawn up according to theories of Chinese medicine.

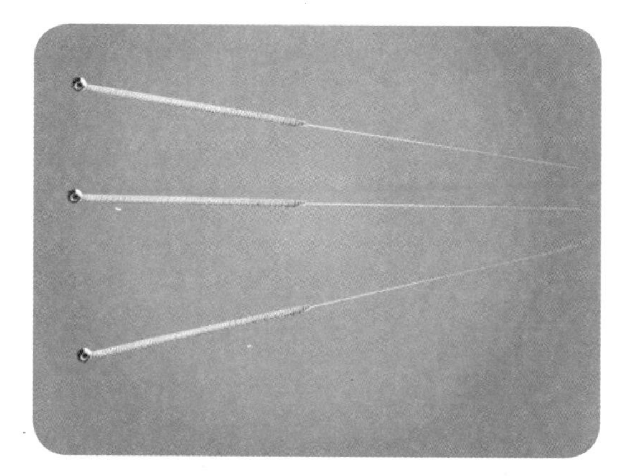

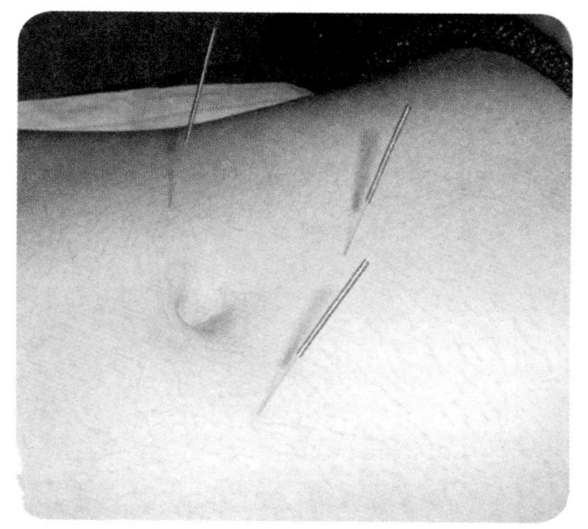

The practitioner will then decide which modality (needles, moxa, cupping, etc.) to use during the present treatment. Usually, needling is performed and often one or more additional treatment modalities are used. The number and location of the needles is decided by the acupuncturist and will probably vary from treatment to treatment, though some points will remain the same and begin to feel familiar. The points that remain the same are usually for the underlying root condition, while the points that change frequently are often to deal with whatever symptoms are most serious at the time of treatment. The amount of needles is not set and can be as few as two or three or as many as thirty, but usually is around ten to fifteen. Needles are mainly placed on the abdomen, back and limbs, with points on the scalp and face also used from time to time, especially for headache. Needle depth is determined by the specific points, since the amount of flesh is different throughout the body. For example, the wrist contains almost no flesh, whereas the thigh contains several inches of muscle. The length of needles is also decided by the acupuncturist and normally ranges between 1.5 - 4.5 cm (0.5 - 1.5 in.).

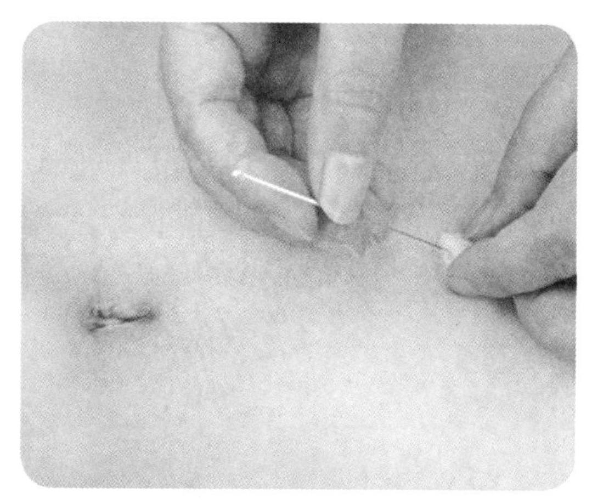

Filiform needles are inserted quickly at an angle of 15 to 90 degrees in relation to the skin's surface. When an experienced acupuncturist inserts the needles, you normally will not feel pain. The sensation is at most like being bitten by an ant. Acupuncture needles are much finer than hypodermic needles used in clinics and hospitals. But most importantly, trained acupuncturists can insert the needles quickly and correctly without causing unnecessary discomfort.

Once the needle has been inserted, one or more of the manipulation techniques mentioned above may be used. The technique used will depend on the disease that is being treated and the practitioner's style of treatment. The patient is supposed to get a specific sensation called *"dé qì"*. This is a sensation specific to acupuncture treatment and literally means "obtaining the qi". The exact feeling varies with each individual. It is usually not pain but a unique sensation of soreness, heaviness, distension, or radiation in some direction. It is generally believed that the stronger the *dé qì* sensation is, the more effective the acupuncture treatment will be. After a few treatments, patients usually start to enjoy this sensation because it is both pleasant and they know the good results it brings. Plus, as stated earlier in explaining how acupuncture works, your brain may begin releasing endorphins, which elicit a sort of natural feeling of well-being.

During treatment, it is best to relax and move as little as possible, unless the practitioner asks you to. Too much movement might cause the needles to bend or become stuck, making them difficult to remove. These accidents are very rare, but if anything happens, stay calm and let the practitioner remove the needles immediately.

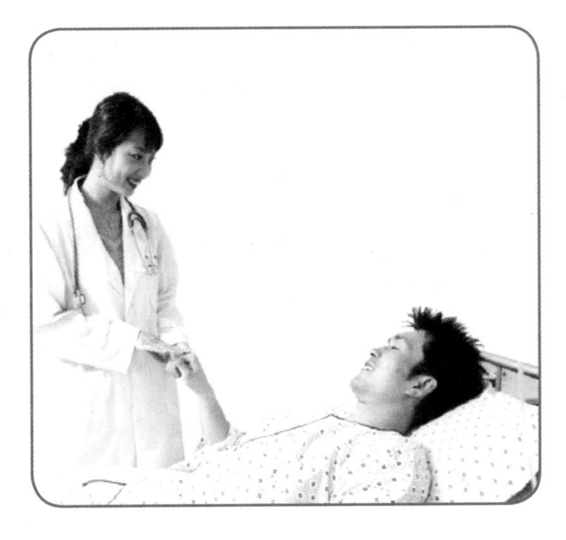

After the needles are inserted, the patient is usually left to relax for about thirty minutes. Other techniques such as moxa or cupping can be performed before or after needling, depending on the situation. After the needles are removed, rise slowly and carefully. There is normally no bleeding during or after acupuncture treatment. If bleeding occurs, it will only be a few drops due to the breakage of small capillaries. Bruising is also very rare, but sometimes happens due to subcutane-

ous bleeding also from broken capillaries. Your practitioner can address any concern before you leave.

After treatment, you will probably feel relaxed and energized. Some of your symptoms may disappear instantly. You may sleep better, have a more regulated appetite, feel less pain, or experience less anxiety.

In rare cases, a patient will be over responsive to the treatment. This usually occurs when a patient is extremely hungry, weak, overtly nervous, or the stimulation and *dé qì* sensation is too strong. The patient might experience nausea, possibly vomiting, develop a very pale complexion, feel weak, sweat excessively, or even faint. If this happens, the acupuncturist will remove all the needles and allow the patient to lie down and rest for a while. Normally the patient will recover quickly. If the patient still feels unwell, a few points may be needled that will help relieve the patient's symptoms.

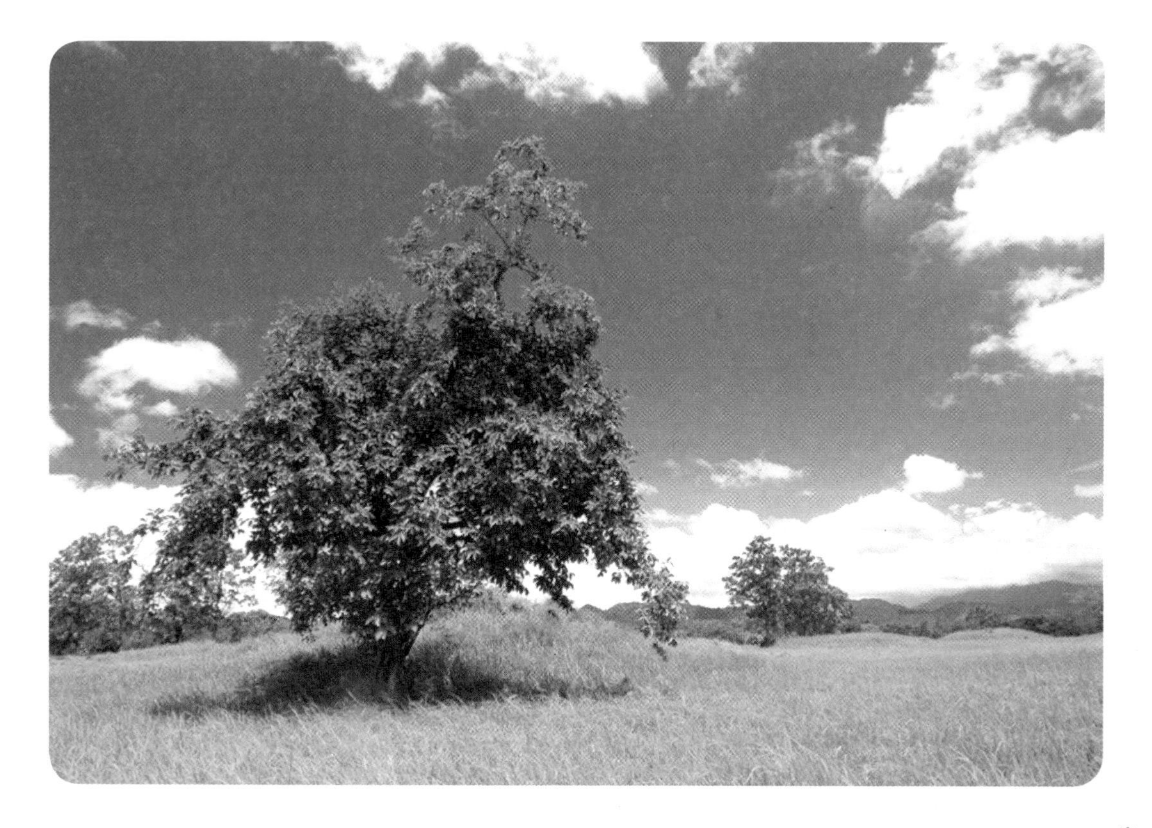

It is advised to be in the best condition possible given your medical situation when you have acupuncture treatment. Don't arrive for your treatment very hungry or just after a large meal, and try to be rested. Also, never arrive after drinking or intoxicated in any way. Intoxicants "scatter" qi and it is impossible for the acupuncturist to balance your body if the qi is thus unstable. Get the most out of your treatment by being extra careful of your general health the day before and after treatment. Help Chinese medicine help you.

3. Treatment Course and Expectations

A typical treatment course will be a couple of visits to the acupuncture clinic per week for a month or two. After this the practitioner and patient will re-evaluate and decide on future treatment. Since migraines are a chronic disease, treatment may take several months.

Even though most patients begin to feel some relief after the first few treatments, Chinese medical treatment is working on a very deep level and to effect lasting change, ample time must be given. The journey to health with Chinese medicine is like everything else in the natural world, there will be ups and downs, times of rapid growth and times of hibernation. With commitment and good communication between practitioner and patient, the journey can be life changing.

4. Translated Research

❶A study was conducted in Sichuan, China in 2007 to explore the differences between electroacupuncture (EA) and biomedical medication for the treatment of migraine headaches due to hyperactivity of liver-yang. 150 cases were assigned to a EA treatment group and a control group. The treatment group was treated with EA at *tài yáng* and the control group received oral administration of biomedical pharmaceuticals. Changes of the score for headache intensity, remission degree of headache, and remission rate of headache after treatment were investigated. After one treatment, VAS score for headache intensity showed dynamic decrease in the control group; in the treatment group the score reached its lowest point 3 - 4 hours after treatment, with the decreasing degree better than the control group. The lasting time for headache remission was significantly longer in the treatment group than that of the control group. So the study showed that EA at *tài yáng* has a transient pain relieving effect for migraine headaches due to hyperactivity of liver-yang, which is comparable to that of routine biomedicine[28].

❷A study in Zhejiang, China, in 2007 was conducted to observe the effects of specific needling techniques used to alleviate

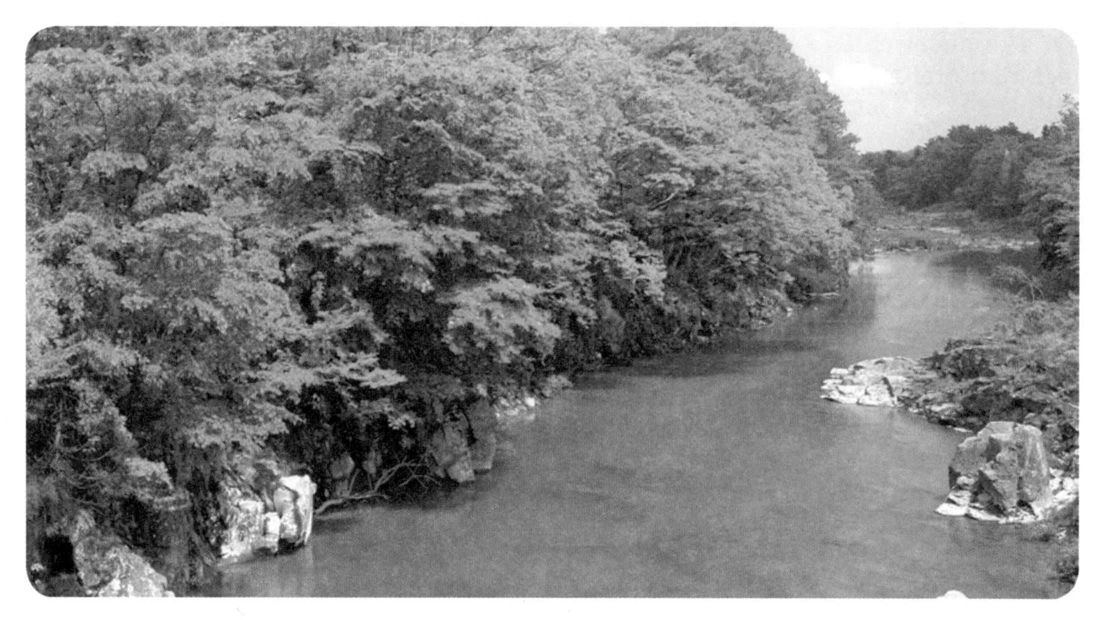

acute stage migraine pain due to blood stasis. The study took 100 patients divided into three groups randomly. Group A received the twisting and shaking method of needle manipulation; Group B received common acupuncture without stimulation; Group C participants were given propyphenazone tablets. Results showed that Group A's rate of recovery was 74%, with 100% of patients experiencing some effect. Group B's rate of recovery was 27%, with 100% of patients experiencing some effect. Group C's rate of recovery was 13%, with 67% of patients experiencing some effect. The study concluded that needle manipulation methods affect the treatment outcome and in particular, the twisting and shaking methods were superior to non-stimulated acupuncture needles. The study also determined that acupuncture is a better treatment therapy for migraines than propyphenazone tablets[30].

❸ A study in Beijing, China, in 2006 observed the curative effects of electroacupuncture and ear acupuncture on migraine headaches. The method involved 90 patients with migraine headaches randomly divided into two treatment groups of 45 persons each. One group was treated with electroacupuncture and ear acupuncture, and the control group treated with flunarizine hydrochloride capsules orally. The result showed the total effective rate of the acupuncture treatment group was 98% and that of the oral medication group was 82%. This study shows that therapy which combines electroacupuncture and ear acupuncture has a better curative effect than oral flunarizine hydrochloride capsules[31].

❹A study was conducted in Shanghai, China, in 2006 to investigate the curative effect of acupuncture on migraines. The study took 205 migraine headache patients and treated them with electroacupuncture and a three-edged needle. The result was compared with a control group that took a biomedical pharmaceutical. The result was a total effective rate of 90% in the acupuncture group and 75% in the control group. Thus, electroacupuncture plus three-edged needle therapy proved more effective than biomedical treatment in this case[32].

❺A study in Zhejiang, China, in 2004 investigated the curative effects of acupuncture on migraine headaches versus oral drug therapy. 186 patients were randomly divided into an acupuncture group and a biomedicine group. The acupuncture group received acupuncture on the nape of the neck and surrounding tissue while the biomedicine group received ergotamine, caffeine and nimodipine. The results showed that the effective rate was 94% in the acupuncture group and 75% in the biomedicine group. In this study, the curative effect of acupuncture was better than that of this drug combination for migraine headaches[33].

❻A study in Guangzhou, China, in 2003 observed the clinical effects of acupuncture on migraine patients with an absence of aura, using three temporal acupuncture points. The method consisted of 62 patients randomly divided into two groups. One group received acupuncture, while the others were treated with nimodipine as a control. The result showed that in the acupuncture group, 13 cases experienced some relief, 10 cases had excellent recovery, and 5 cases had total recovery, with the total effective rate 80%. In the nimodipine group, 4 cases experienced some recovery, 3 cases had excellent recovery, while 8 cases had total recovery. The total effective rate for the drug group equaled 56%, showing that the curative effect of acupuncture is better than that of the drug nimodipine[34].

❼A study in Hebei, China, in 2002 observed the treatment of acupuncture and oxygen therapy for migraine headaches. 128 persons received acupuncture combined with O_2 therapy versus another 128 persons in a control group treated by routine prescription medication. Observations recorded therapeutic effects and side-effects. Results showed the total effective rate was 100% in the acupuncture - O_2 treatment group, and 84% in the non-acupuncture group. Significant difference between the two groups was also noted in relation to side-effects. In conclusion, acupuncture combined with O_2 therapy is an ideal method to treat migraines due to its high cure rate and minimal side-effects[35].

Chinese Medicinals

1. What Are Chinese Medicinals?

❶ Introduction

As early as 4,000 years ago, the ancestors of the Chinese people created primitive medicine in their struggle with nature and disease. When searching for and gathering food, they soon understood that some plant, animal, and mineral substances could relieve or even eliminate some diseases. This was the origin of the development and application of Chinese herbal medicine.

In time, clinical and anecdotal experience using different substances developed into a sophisticated system of choosing medicinal substances based on the identification of complex patterns rather than merely based on symptoms. This system is based on categorizing substances by their inherent nature and tastes. It also details which organs are affected by an individual herb or a formulation of herbs.

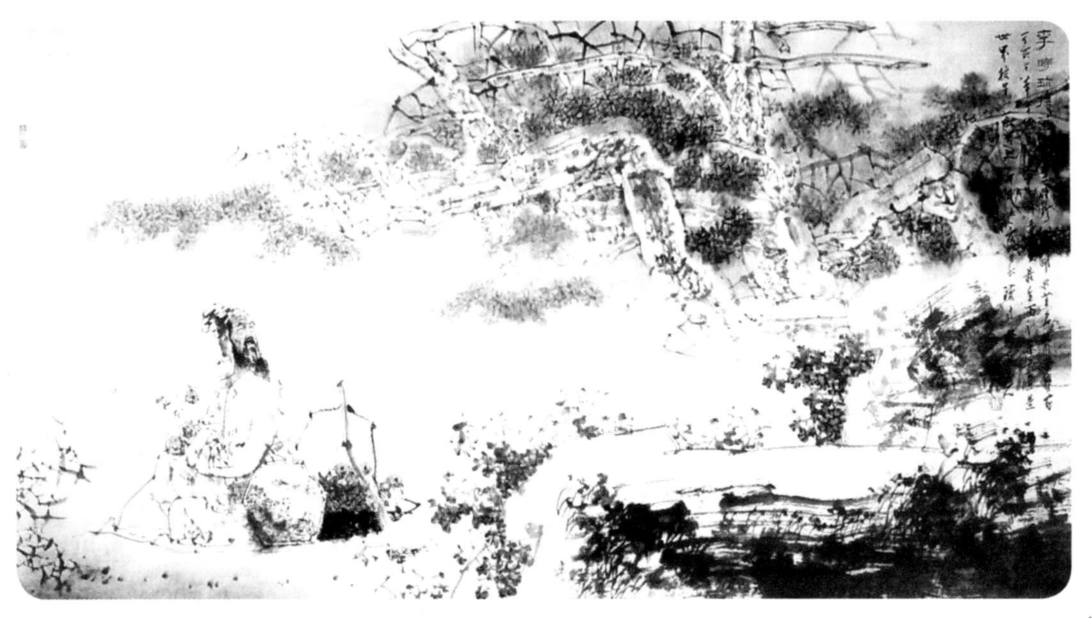

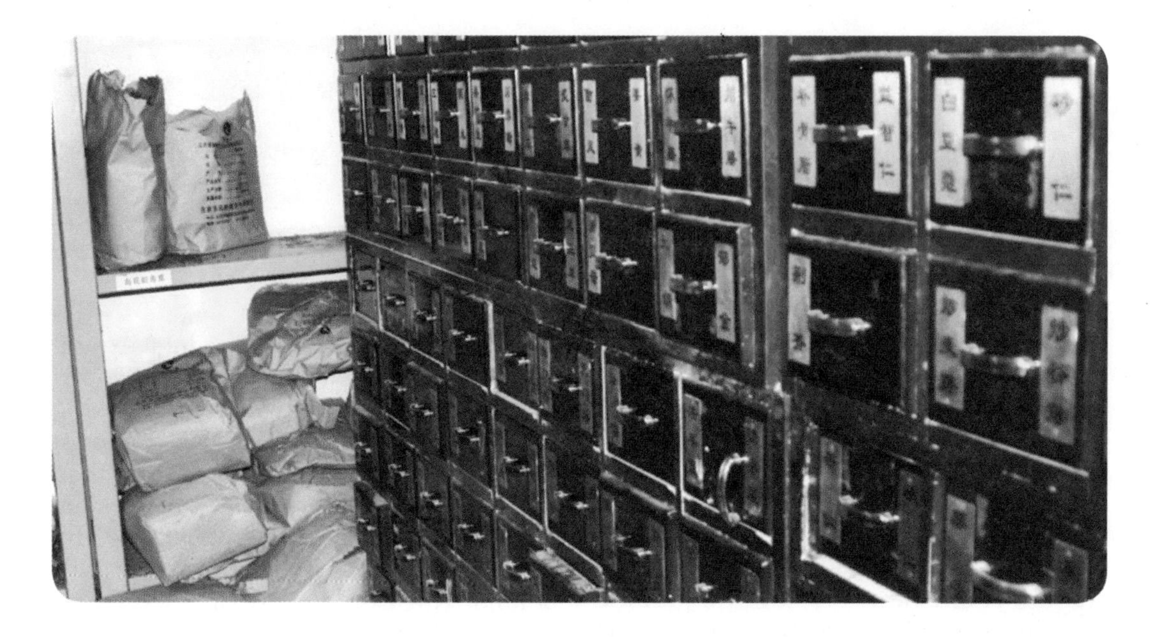

Centuries of documentation have given us a wealth of detailed information today about medicinal combinations. In fact, hundreds of formulations perfected decades, centuries or even millennia ago are still commonly used today with their original ingredients because they have been found to be so effective. Yet the best therapy is always tailored to the individual patient. Using the entire system of Chinese medicine, an experienced doctor can treat each patient uniquely and devise a specific prescription for each problem.

The phrase "Chinese Medicinal" refers to substances that occur naturally in the environment and can come from plant, animal, or mineral sources. Today it is increasingly called "organic medicine" to differentiate it from chemical pharmaceutical products which are generally constructed from specific chemical molecules rather than natural whole substances. These medicinals can be prepared in a variety of ways in order to be used by the body. Chinese medicinals can be drunk, eaten, inhaled, or applied to the skin. They regulate the body's qi, blood, yin, yang, and expel pathogens as well. There are over 3,000 thousand different substances listed in ancient pharmacology books, though only about 400 or so are commonly used. In fact, any natural substance on earth can be used in Chinese medicine, but it will only be called a Chinese medicinal when it is used according to the theories and construct of Chinese medicine.

❷ Mechanism of Chinese medicinals

The underlying idea between how Chinese medicinals work is fundamentally different than that behind biomedical pharmaceuticals. A pharmaceutical is a finely crafted and intensely focused creation. Years, sometimes decades, of research occurs before any drug is released on the market. The chemists and scientists strive to isolate the exact chemical or combination of chemicals that can cause a very specific change in some bodily functions. The change elicited by these drugs is often effective at relieving symptoms, but rarely restores the damaged body part or function whose breakdown was responsible for the symptoms in the first place. For example, antibiotics will kill invading bacteria, but will not strengthen the body against further invasions; or a pain killer may relieve the aching joints of an arthritis patient, but it will not stop or even retard the progression of the disease. In addition, it is not uncommon for a drug to cause unwanted side-effects along with its desired actions. Biomedical drugs may damage the nervous system, the digestive system, or most commonly, the liver or kidneys.

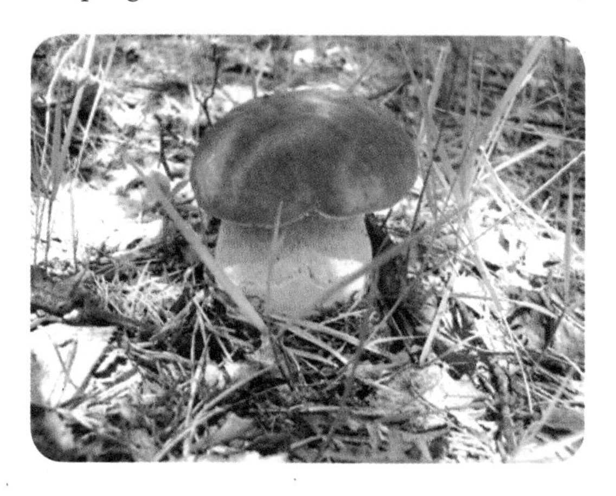

In Chinese medicine, as mentioned above, the idea is to restore the body's innate ability to remain in a state of health. In severe cases, long term treatment is necessary to provide constant support to the body, but usually patients who start treatment with Chinese medicine are able to stop treatment after their symptoms have been brought under control. Treatment is able to be stopped because the medicine used was helping to restore the body's damaged functions, not just as a substitute. These patients then gladly use the principles of Chinese medicine throughout their lives to maintain health, only visiting an acupuncturist or herbalist to take care of any health problems that appear as a natural result of aging.

To a doctor of Chinese medicine, negative side-effects are a sign of improper treatment, either due to faulty diagnosis, or inappropriate treatment methods. A properly constructed herbal formula will exactly match the patient's internal patterns and will cause little if any kind of other imbalance. What is weak will be strengthened, what is too strong will be reigned in, leaving no room for other problems to develop due to the ingredients of the prescription. It is commonly thought that because Chinese medicinals include the whole biological substance, as opposed to an artificially isolated biologically active constituent, the naturally occurring ingredients that make up the harmonious living organism help to buffer the body from side-effects. Here is an analogy. Taking vitamin pills can help to quickly supplement nutrients you need. Yet they cannot replace food, a mixture of necessary nutrients and "unnecessary" substances, for the long-term maintenance of health. So is the case with synthesized drugs. Many of them are extracted from plants. They are effective and helpful. But most cannot replace natural medicinals, a mixture of effective ingredients and unidentified or "ineffective" ingredients, for the long-term treatment of chronic diseases.

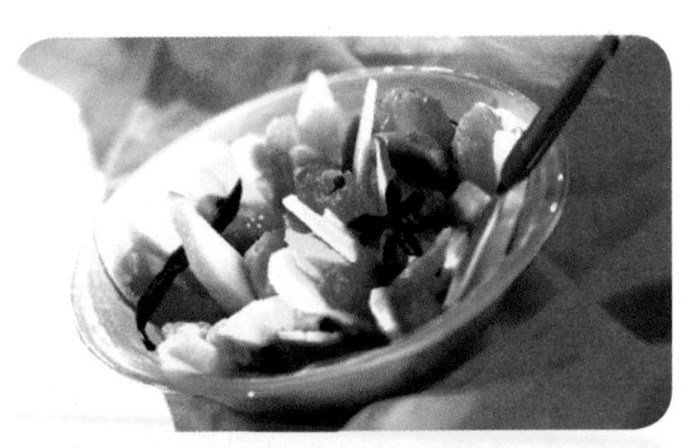

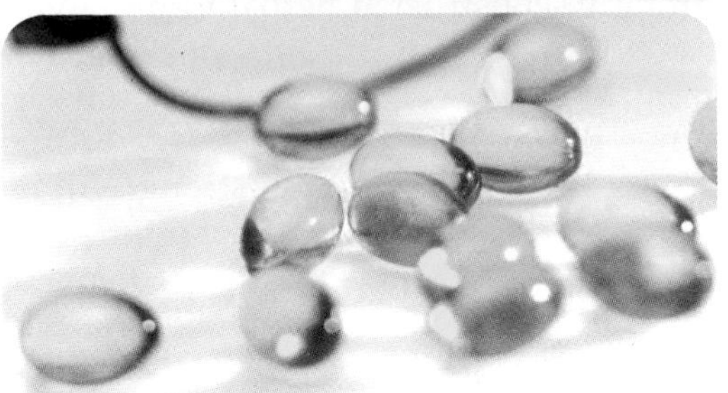

Another mechanism that makes Chinese medicinals safe is that they are counterbalanced within the formula. As an example, medicinals that take out excess heat from the body are considered cold, and can damage the digestive system. Therefore, in many formulas that treat excess heat, a couple of medicinals that promote and strengthen digestion may be added. If the patient has weak digestion to begin with, even more ingredients are reserved for that purpose. This kind of treatment is much more than simply anti-symptomatic. Each prescription must be a balanced entity, which perfectly compliments the patient's condition. When used properly, Chinese medicinals are safe and effective. This takes experience and active involvement by the practitioner. Sound and individualized diagnosis is made based on the patient's present condition to ensure efficacy and safety.

❸ Classification of medicinals

Every medicinal substance has unique properties including a nature that can be warm, cool, or neutral; one or more tastes that include sour, bitter, sweet, acrid, or salty; and several functions. Proper selection of medicinals is the key to avoiding side-effects. As they say, "One man's meat is another's poison."

A medicinal's nature and tastes reveal how it affects the body. For example, since coptis is cold and bitter, it is used to drain heat syndromes that are causing symptoms like thirst, mouth ulcers, constipation, or a yellow tongue coating. Cold medicinals are used for heat syndromes, and the bitter taste drains downward, so a cold and bitter medicinal is said to drain heat from the body. Medicinals also focus on certain organs or areas of the body. Coptis has an affinity to the heart, so it is often used for heat patterns in the heart. Another bitter and cold medicinal, scutellaria, has an affinity to the lungs, so is used differently than coptis, despite having the same nature and taste.

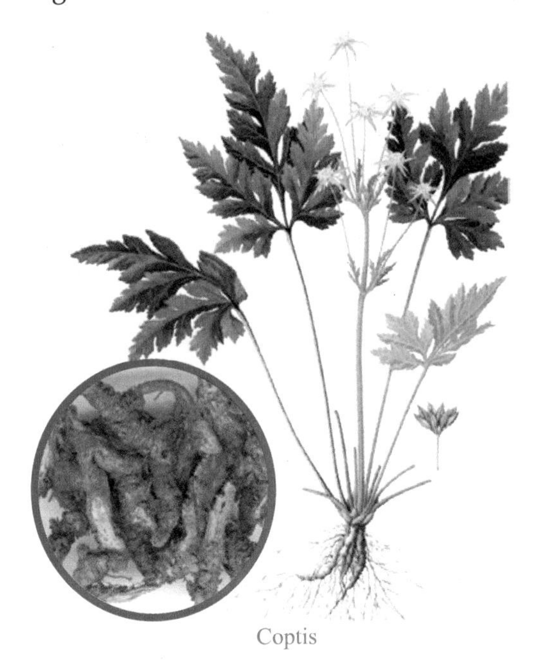

Coptis

The selection of the medicinal is made according to the pattern identified. If a patient presents with signs of qi deficiency like shortness of breath, fatigue, lack of energy, weak pulse, and a pale tongue, medicinals that supplement qi will be added. If signs of yin deficiency are obvious such as emaciation, feeling hot in the afternoon, night sweats, irritability, a fine pulse, and a thin tongue with little coating, medicals that supplement yin will be administered. In clinical practice, practitioners of Chinese medicine gradually form a number of basic formulas that fit the common patterns seen in each disease. These formulas will be modified according to each specific case.

Current research scientists have investigated the mechanism behind some of the medicinals used in the treatment of migraine headaches. In a recent review it was shown that the effects of medicinals commonly used in the treatment of migraine headaches have several different mechanisms depending on the substance. For example, the major component of notopterygium can stop the sensation of pain in animal experiments. Other medicinals and formulas have also been found to have effects through different avenues. Although a clearer and more complete pictures of their mechanisms are warranted, it is obvious that Chinese medicinals can contribute to the successful management of migraine headaches in the clinic.

④ Compatibility of medicinals

Ancient people called the relationships between medicinals "seven modes of emotion". Among these methods, the first one is "single medicine". The "single medicine" method is when treatment uses only one Chinese medicinal substance. Generally speaking, this method fits simple acute disorders, or early childhood conditions. One simple problem gets one simple substance. This method is convenient, effective and fitting for certain disorders, but is rarely used in clinical practice, as most conditions that are seen in clinic are more complex. However, this method might be used when other options are not available, such as when traveling.

When the condition is complicated, a single medicinal cannot treat the whole person effectively, because it cannot address or distinguish between primary and secondary problems, and cannot give real consideration to multiple signs and symptoms. In these situations, two or more substances are necessary to treat the condition. When medicinals are combined, one substance can impact the other. That impact may promote or degrade the action of either substance, or it may restrain or eliminate any toxicity. Rarely, two or more ingredients together can possibly produce toxicity or adverse reactions where there was none when the medicinals were used individually. Chinese herbal medicine has been created through centuries of clinical experience and close patient observation.

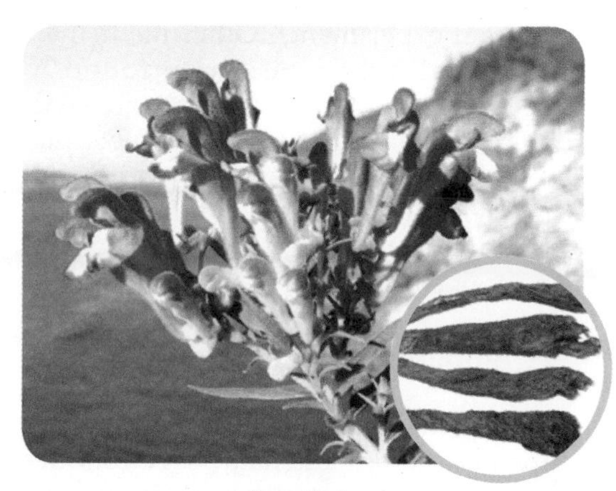

Scutellaria

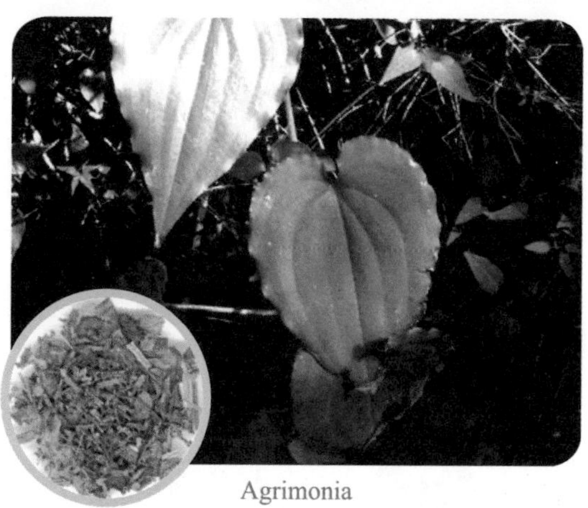

Agrimonia

When two or more medicinals are used at the same time, close attention must be paid to the results. These interactions have been summarized into six different kinds. These are mutual promotion, mutual toxicity, mutual restraint, mutual detoxification, mutual inhibition, and mutual opposition. These are simply explained by the following four aspects of medicinal compatibility: some medicines can produce synergistic effects to increase their effective properties; the efficiency of some medicines can be diminished when they are combined; intrinsic toxic properties can be relieved by combinations; and some medicinals can become toxic in combination even though they are harmless when used singly. From these complex and well-defined rules, one can see that formulas are composed of medicinals according to certain rules of compatibility and dosage for both safety and maximum efficacy.

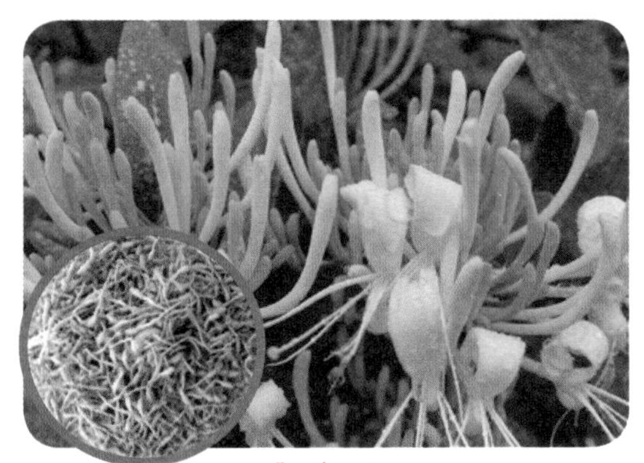

Lonicera

❺ Commonly used medicinals

Chinese medicinals are very rarely used alone. But in order to construct a proper formula, the practitioner must be familiar with the properties of each individual substance. Since patients may present in any possible combination of patterns, any one of the thousands of medicinal substances may show up in a patient's formula. But as we have seen, there are a few main patterns that typically present in a migraine headache patient. And for each of these main patterns, there are certain medicinals that are most effective and therefore most commonly used. In addition, due to clinical and laboratory research, some herbs are known to be more effective in the treatment of migraines than others. Below are some brief descriptions of some of the most commonly used medicinals to treat this painful and debilitating disorder:

Borneol 冰片 *Bīng piàn* (Broneolum Syntheticum)

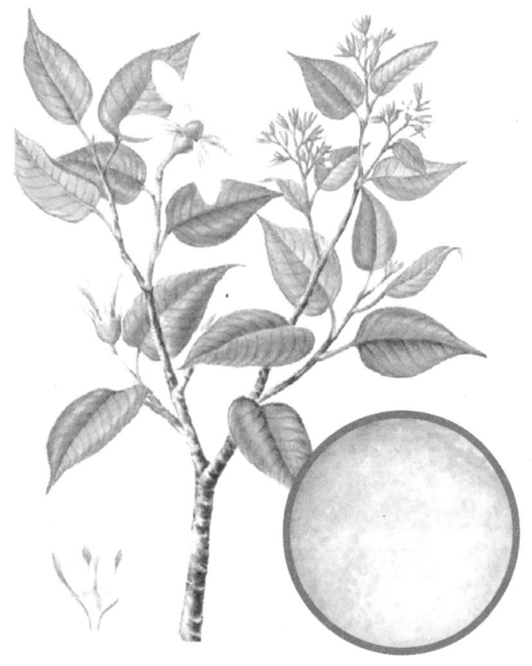

Borneol

Source: Camphor Tree Crystals
Properties: acrid, bitter, slightly cold

Bīng piàn means "Ice Slice" and is used for heat syndromes. It's fragrant smell is used to awaken patients from unconsciousness, clear heat, relieve swelling and stop pain. It is often used in formulas that are designed to be applied to the skin. Patients with rising liver yang will feel cool and soothed when *bīng piàn* is applied to the forehead, temples, or back of the neck.

Bīng piàn applied to the skin has been shown to cause slight numbness, stop pain and have antiseptic qualities. It can also pass through the blood-brain barrier within five minutes, with lasting cumulative effects on the brain.

Notoptetygium Root and Rhizome 羌活 *Qiāng huó* (Rhizomza Seu Radix Notopterygii)

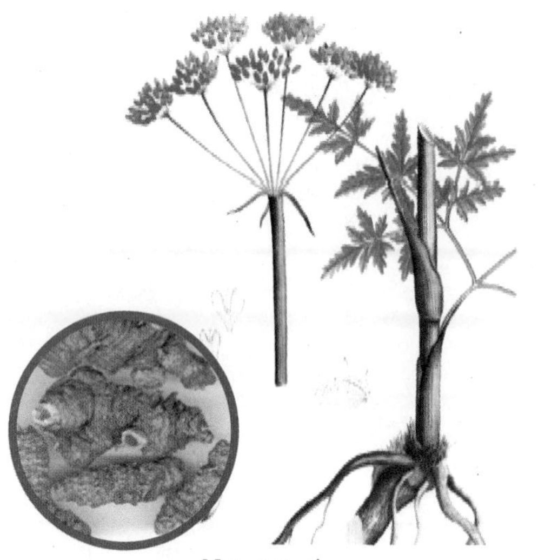

Notoptetygium

Source: Notoptetygium Root and Rhizome
Properties: bitter, acrid, slightly warm

Qiāng huó is one of two plants with the character *huó* 活 in their name that are used to treat pain. The effect of *qiāng huó* focuses on the upper body, expelling exterior cold, dampness and wind to relax the joints and stop pain. It is mainly used in the upper body for problems affecting the neck, head and shoulders. The other *huó* is used for the lower back and legs. In Chinese, 活 means "alive" or "active" and reveals the activating power in *qiāng huó*. The acrid flavor also indicates that this substance can invigorate qi and expel stagnant cold and dampness that obstruct the channels and cause pain. Patients who experience stiff neck and shoulders or inflammation/swelling in the upper extremities, neck and head along with their headaches will often be treated with *qiāng huó*.

Qiāng huó has been shown to lower cerebrovascular blood flow when combined with other medicinals.

Chuanxiong 川芎 *Chuān xiōng* (Rhizoma Chuanxiong)

Source: Chuanxiong Rhizome
Properties: bitter, acrid, warm

Chuān xiōng is possibly the single most used herb for headache in Chinese medicine. It promotes blood and qi flow throughout the body, eliminates wind to stop pain, and treats many diseases due to

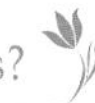

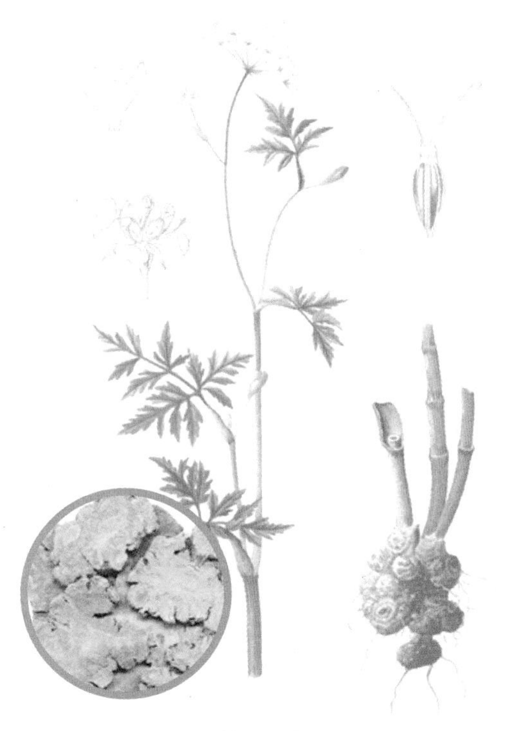
Chuan xiong

blood stagnation. This includes irregular menstruation, amenorrhea, abdominal pain due to intestinal obstruction, chest or rib side pain, and pain from traumatic injuries. It specifically treats wind-dampness type headaches.

Chuān xiōng can dilate blood vessels and relieve vascular smooth muscle spasms. *Chuān xiōng* crosses the blood-brain barrier and also inhibits the formation of clots to improve microcirculation.

Chinese Lovage 藁本 *Gāo běn* (Rhizoma Ligustici)

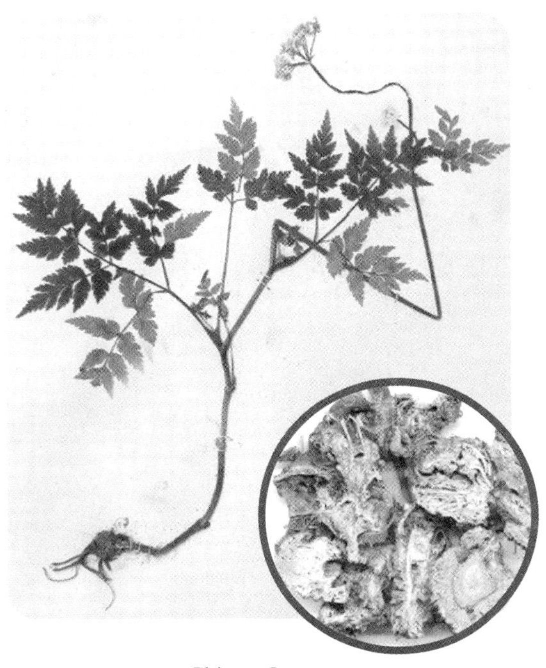
Chinese Lovage

Source: Chinese Lovage Rhizome
Properties: fragrant, bitter, acrid

Gāo běn expels wind, cold, and dampness to treat the common cold and arthritic types of joint pain. It also treats headaches that are accompanied with digestive disorders such as abdominal pain, diarrhea, and intestinal obstructions, or scaly eruptions on the scalp.

Gāo běn has been shown by research to have a moderate pain-relieving effect.

Long Pepper 荜茇 *Bì bá*
(Fructus Piperis Longi)

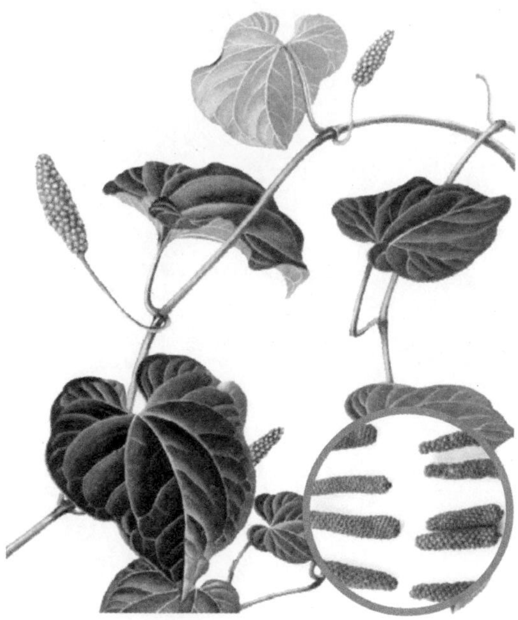

Long Pepper

Source: Immature Long Pepper
Properties: acrid, hot

Because it is hot and spicy, *bì bá* can expel stubborn, lingering cold in the intestines and stomach, warm the spleen and stomach, and stop pain. This warming function also relieves nausea, vomiting and diarrhea. Aside from stomach disorders *bì bá* can also treat toothache when used externally. Formulas that contain *bì bá* benefit from its sedative and convulsion-relieving effects to help relieve migraine symptoms.

The essential oil of *bì bá* can reinforce the capability of standing oxygen deficiency, dilate blood vessels for heart ischemia and lower blood pressure which could alleviate hepertension-related migraines significantly. This essential oil also resists bacteria and viruses.

Salvia 丹参 *Dān shēn*
(Radix Salviae Miltiorrhiae)

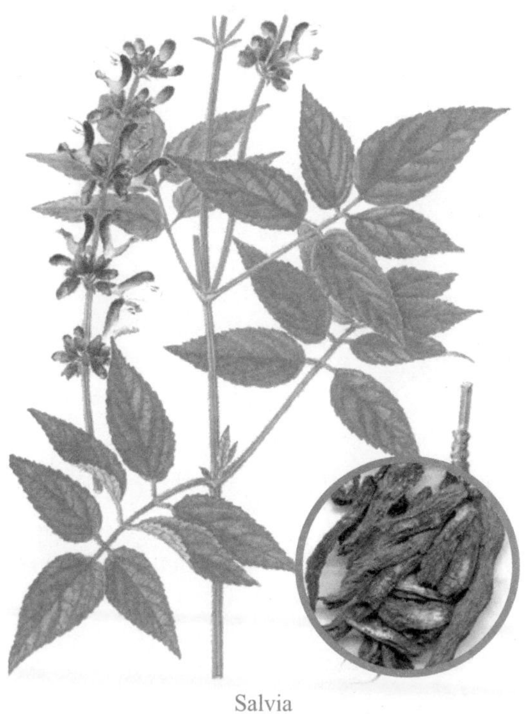

Salvia

Source: Salvia Root
Properties: bitter, slightly cold

Dān shēn is prescribed for an array of disorders from irregular menstruation, menorrhea, intestinal bloating or obstruction, prickling chest and abdominal pain, to rheumatoid arthritis and other types of swelling and pain due to an enlarged liver or spleen. For migraines, this medicinal helps to eliminate long-standing blood stasis to cure the root of the disease.

The effective component of *dān shēn* can increase blood flow through the coronary arteries, reduce blood cholesterol and viscosity, and resist platelet agglutination.

Saffron 藏红花 *Zàng hóng huā* (Stigma Croci)

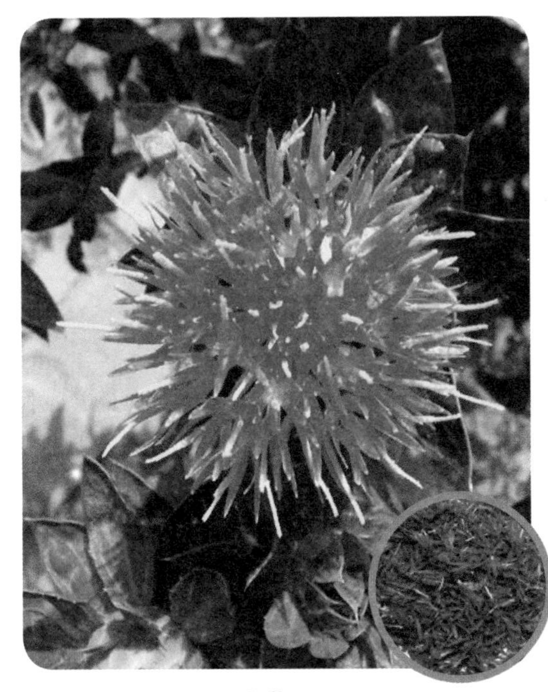

Saffron

Source: Saffron Stigma
Properties: sweet, slightly bitter, cold

Zàng hóng huā is used to treat blood stasis. It is used widely for blood problems during menstruation, after childbirth, for injuries, to prevent or treat clots in the arteries, as well as for nervous exhaustion, anxiety and many types of headache. Saffron can be extremely expensive, often at over $10 per gram. Another flower with similar medicinal effects, called carthamus, is often used as an affordable substitute to true saffron.

Modern pharmacology studies show that saffron can improve heart muscle oxygen supply. And due to its glycoside content, it can increase the volume of blood flow in the coronary arteries.

Bupleurum 柴胡 *Chái hú* (Radix Bupleuri)

Source: Bupleurum Root
Properties: bitter, slightly cold

Chái hú, meaning "Kindling of the Barbarians", is used to harmonize the liver. When emotional tension builds up, this often causes the qi of the liver to become stagnant. Since qi is yang, when it is disturbed it often moves upwards, into the head. Headaches from a stagnant liver are often accompanied by alternating feelings of hot and cold, gas pains in the chest and rib side, irregular menstruation, and irritability.

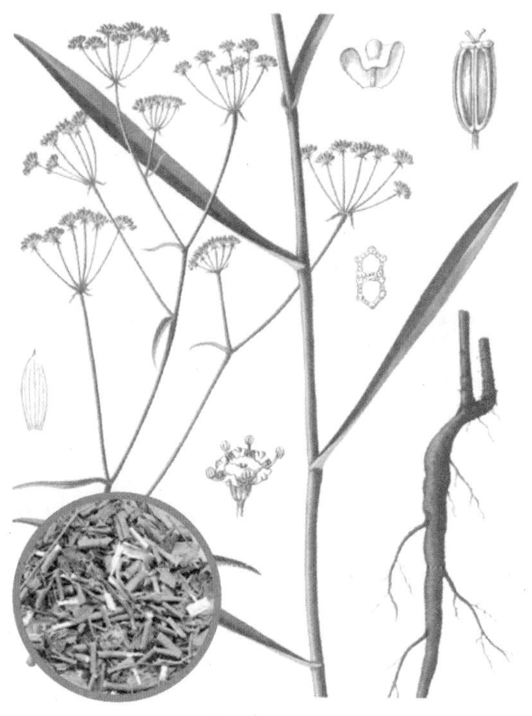

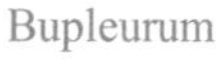
Bupleurum

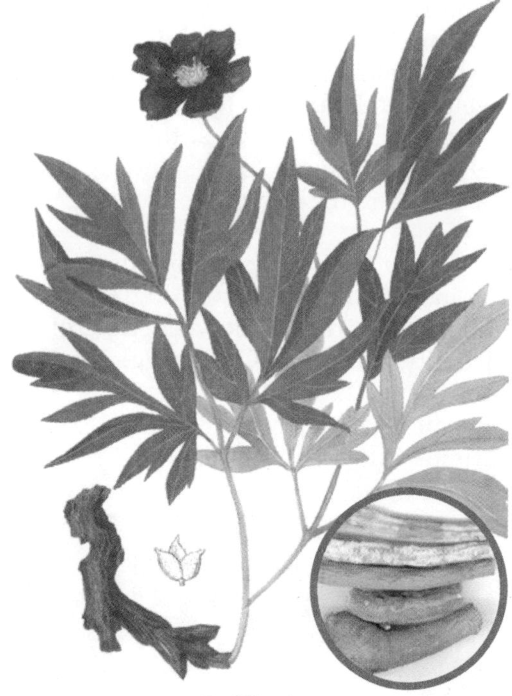

Red Peony

Active components include supersaponin and sapogenin, which can enhance a person's pain threshold and relieve pain.

Red Peony 赤芍 ***Chì sháo***
(Radix Paeoniae Rubra)

Source: Red Peony Root
Properties: bitter, slightly cold

Chì sháo can remove heat to cool blood and eliminate blood stasis by activating blood circulation to stop pain. This herb treats numerous disorders, including infectious diseases like influenza, various bleeding disorders, redness and swelling of the eye, abdominal pain due to intestinal obstruction, injury from trauma and other types of pain.

Chì sháo can expand vessel walls and increase coronary blood flow. Clinically, it has been shown to be effective for treating migraines in combination with other medicinals. It can also restrain the formation of clots in the arteries thereby diminishing risks of stroke or heart attack.

2. What Will Treatment Be Like?

Chinese medicinals are the mainstay of Chinese medicine. Although acupuncture is the best known modality here in the West, in China the great majority of patients who seek treatment from Chinese medicine get medicinal formulas. Treatment with Chinese medicinals is thought to have a wider scope than the more commonly known acupuncture, and for most diseases it works faster. Another, more practical advantage of treatment with Chinese medicinals is the frequency of office visits. Acupuncture patients are frequently seen two or three times per week,

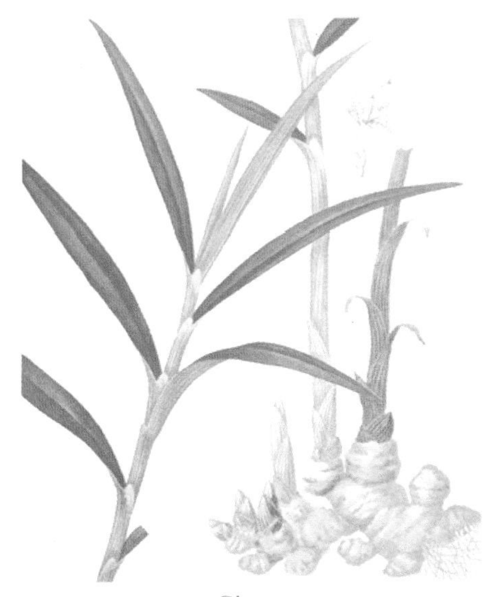
Ginger

while formulas are usually modified once a week, with visits becoming even less frequent as the patient's condition stabilizes.

Similar to the modalities that work on the points and channels like acupuncture, moxibustion, cupping, etc., Chinese medicinals can be administered in many different ways. The most common method in China is done by taking the raw medicinals, boiling them to extract their effective properties, and then drinking the resulting liquid like tea. Chinese medicine calls this a "decoction". In general, taking Chinese medicinals as a decoction is the most potent and fastest working form of treatment available.

Since treatment methods vary greatly from disease to disease, and styles differ between practitioners, the exact dosage, number of packets, and preparation instructions will likewise be very different. Here we are trying to give a general idea about a typical treatment. If your practitioner gives you something that falls outside the guidelines listed here, do not be concerned.

❶ Preparation of the decoction

At the practitioner's office, you will most likely be given several packets of Chinese medicinals. Each packet will be for one or two days use and will probably contain from 70 - 120 grams of herbs. Take the time to examine the herbs in the packet. Enjoy the different colors, smells, and textures. As many Chinese medicinals are common plants found around the world, you may even find something you recognize. Being able to get to know your medicine and the ability to be involved in its preparation is one thing that never fails to endear a patient to Chinese medicine.

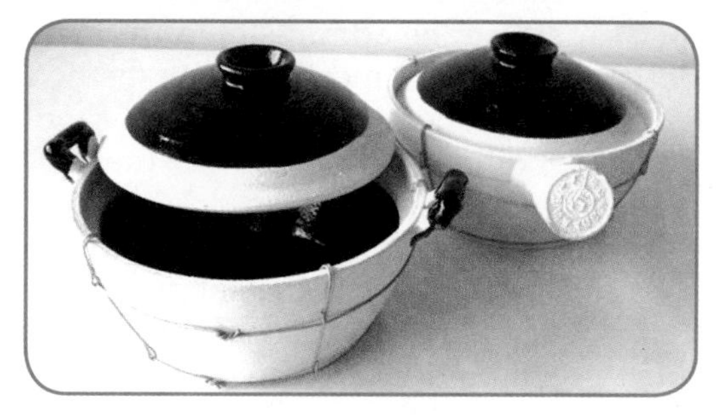

Decoction Pot

To cook the decoction, first put all the medicinals into a ceramic or glass pot (metal is not suitable) and add water until it completely covers the medicinals, or add a specific amount that your practitioner tells you to add. The mixture should be brought to a boil on high heat and then reduced to a medium flame. Usually the decoction needs to be simmered for 20-60 minutes depending on the ingredients of the formula. Strain the decoction, divide the liquid in two, and drink it twice a day in two equal portions, usually once with breakfast and once with dinner. Most often, one packet is one day's dosage. Sometimes you will be asked to save the dregs to be cooked again in the future. In this case, they should be stored in the refrigerator. There are some ingredients that have special cooking instructions such as cooking alone for 20 - 30 minutes before other ingredients are added, for especially dense materials; those that should be added at the last five minutes of cooking, for very delicate medicinals; or those that should be added to the strained decoction after cooking, for materials in powder, gel, or liquid form.

Recently, some clinics offer a decoction cooking service. The decoction will be made by a machine and sealed in plastic

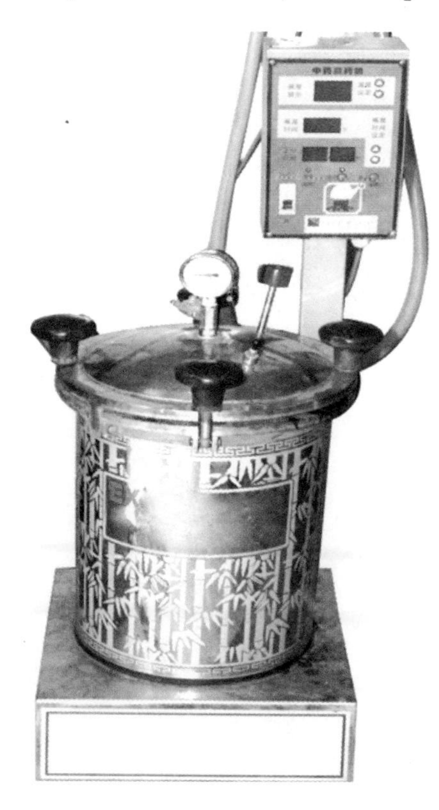

Decoction Machine

bags to store in the refrigerator. No matter if you or the clinic prepares the herbs, when you drink your decoction it should be warm. Only in special cases is room temperature or cooler acceptable. You are advised to take the decoction about one hour before meals. If the decoction irritates your stomach, take it after meals.

At first you may find making your decoction troublesome, and/or have a strong dislike of the unfamiliar taste. This is a common problem, especially in the West where we are accustomed to our medicine being easy to take and either tasteless or sugar coated. We can only ask that you recall the millions of people who have benefited from this treatment method and give a fair trial, at least two weeks, to the decoction method. In fact, it is the experience of many doctors and patients that if the prescription properly fits the imbalance, the initially unfamiliar or unpleasant taste will become something the patient enjoys and looks forward to.

2 Treatment course

For chronic diseases, decoctions take time to have an effect. When you go to the clinic the first time, the practitioner will usually give a prescription for 3 - 7 days. You will need to come back to the clinic about once a week for the practitioner to modify the formula. After a month or so has passed, you and your practitioner will reevaluate your condition and your treatment strategy may change allowing for gradually smaller amounts of medicinals, and more infrequent office visits. A treatment course usually lasts a few months, but may be more or less depending on the severity of the case.

3 Common formulas

A typical formula consists of between 5 to 15 ingredients with each ingredient usually dosed between 3 and 30 grams. The ingredients in the formula are arranged according to a hierarchy. The chief ingredient represents the main therapeutic effect and will often have the largest dose. The assistants and deputies either support the chief, address another aspect of the imbalance, or perform a checking action against some other ingredient that may be too harsh in some way. The last soldier, the courier, serves to guide the formula to a certain body part, organ, or channel, or acts to harmonize the formula. See if you can recognize some of the single herbs mentioned above in the formulas below.

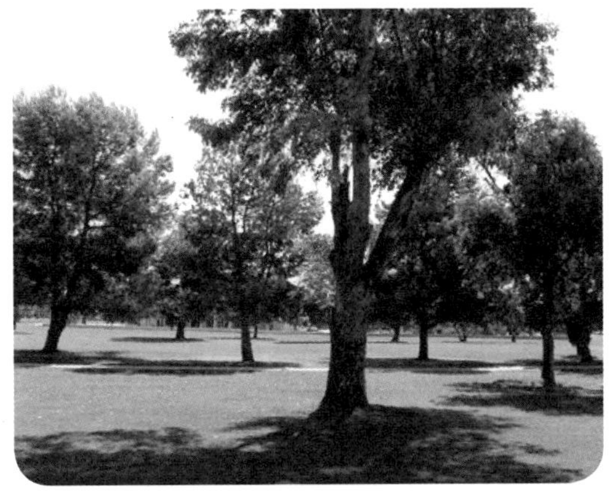

Liver-yang headache

Typical manifestations: headache accompanied by dizziness, restlessness, irritability, rib side pain, and a bitter taste in the mouth.

Treatment Principle: calm the liver and suppress yang

Gastrodia and Uncaria Decoction (*Tiān Má Gōu Téng Yǐn*) 天麻钩藤饮

Common Name	Pinyin	Chinese Name	Latin Name	Dose
Gastrodia rhizome	*Tiān má*	天麻	Rhizoma Gastrodiae	9g
Gardenia fruit	*Zhī zǐ*	栀子	Fructus Gardeniae	9g
Scutellaria root	*Huáng qín*	黄芩	Radix Scutellariae	9g
Eucommia bark	*Dù zhòng*	杜仲	Cortex Eucommiae	9g
Leonurus herb	*Yì mǔ cǎo*	益母草	Herba Leonuri	9g
Mistletoe	*Sāng jì shēng*	桑寄生	Herba Taxilli	9g
Flowery knotwood stem	*Yè jiāo téng*	夜交藤	Caulis Polygoni Multiflori	9g
Root poria	*Fú shén*	茯神	Radix Poriae Pini	9g
Cyathula root	*Chuān niú xī*	川牛膝	Radix Cyathulae	12g
Uncaria stem	*Gōu téng*	钩藤	Ramulus Uncariae Cum Uncis	12g
Abalone Shell	*Shí jué míng*	石决明	Concha Haliotidis	18g

Gastrodia and Uncaria Decoction is one of the most commonly used prescriptions to for migraines due to excessive rising of liver-yang. During migraine treatment, a doctor will likely modify a prescription for the particular signs and as the condition changes. Different medicinals can be used when there is insomnia or severe pain, and also to focus the formula on a particular aspect of the head, such as the forehead or the back of the head[36].

Blood deficiency headache

Typical manifestations: headache accompanied by dizziness, a pale complexion, heart palpitations, and a pale tongue.

Treatment Principle: supplement and nourish qi and blood

Four Ingredients Decoction (*Sì Wù Tāng*) 四物汤

Common Name	Pinyin	Chinese Name	Latin Name	Dose
Rehmannia root	*Shú dì huáng*	熟地	Radix Rehmanniae Praeparata	15g
Chinese angelica root	*Dāng guī*	当归	Radix Angelicae Sinensis	15g
White peony root	*Bái sháo*	白芍	Radix Paeoniae Alba	10g
Chuanxiong rhizome	*Chuān xiōng*	川芎	Rhizoma Chuanxiong	8g

Four Ingredients Decoction is a nearly 1,000 year old formula and is one of the most commonly used in Chinese medicine. Traditionally this formula, or a modified version, was used to treat nearly every type of women's disease. But in the past few years with greater research into its effects, its uses have expanded. In the clinic, peach kernel and carthamus can be added to treat migraine headaches due to blood deficiency[37].

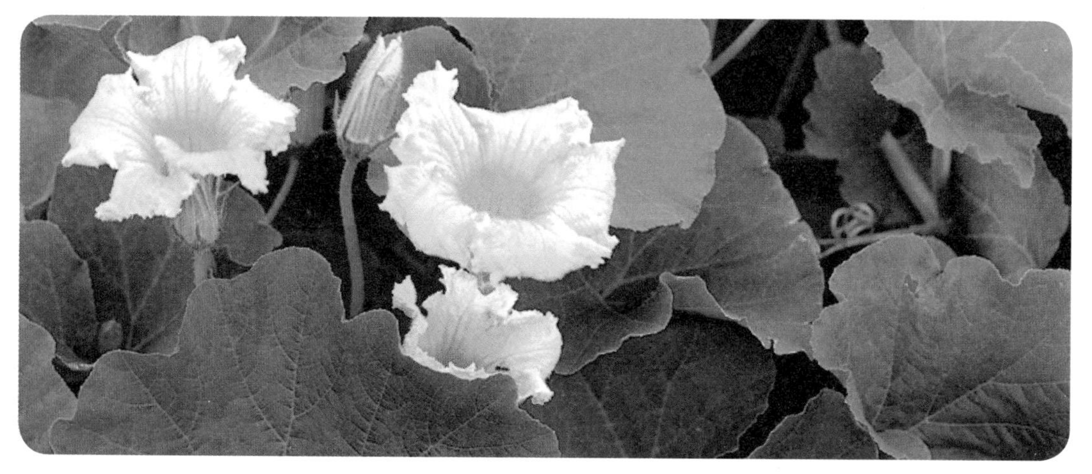

Phlegm turbidity headache

Typical manifestations: headache accompanied by dizziness, vomiting, nausea, and a greasy tongue coating.

Treatment Principle: transform phlegm and descend counterflow qi

Pinellia, Atractylodes and Gastrodia Decoction (*Bàn Xià Bái Zhū Tiān Má Tāng*) 半夏白术天麻汤

Common Name	Pinyin	Chinese Name	Latin Name	Dose
Phellodendron bark	*Huáng bǎi*	黄柏	Cortex Phellodendri	6 g
Dried ginger	*Gān jiāng*	干姜	Rhizoma Zingiberis	9 g
Gastrodia rhizome	*Tiān má*	天麻	Rhizoma Gastrodiae	15 g
Atractylodes rhizome	*Cāng zhú*	苍术	Rhizoma Atractylodis	15 g
Poria fungus	*Fú líng*	茯苓	Poria	15 g
Astragalus root	*Huáng qí*	黄芪	Radix Astragali	15 g
Alisma rhizome	*Zé xiè*	泽泻	Rhizoma Alismatis	15 g
Ginseng root	*Rén shēn*	人参	Radix et Rhizoma Ginseng	15 g
White atractylodis	*Bái zhú*	白术	Rhizoma Atractylodis Macrocephalae	3 g
Medicated laven	*Shén qū*	神曲	Massa Medicata Fermentata	3 g
Pinellia Rhizome	*Bàn xià*	半夏	Rhizoma Pinelliae	15 g
Tangerine peel	*Jú pí*	橘皮	Pericarpium Citri Reticulatae	15 g

This prescription is one of the most commonly used to clear phlegm and turbidity in the body. "Phlegm" in Chinese medicine is characterized by heaviness, excess mucus such as in sinus obstruction and cough, and an overweight body. Phlegm may occur when there are deficient fluids, which causes vessels to dry up and blood to thicken.

A high level of "bad" cholesterol is a phlegm condition because it causes thick, sticky blood. Or it could come from excess dampness, which eventually becomes thicker and heavier and clogs vital passageways. Qi deficiency may also cause phlegm by degrading the digestive system where food and nutrients are not properly processed. Phlegm can block any organ, but is particularly prone to small openings such as in the chest, face, head and heart. When patients have dizziness, chest distress, and a thick and greasy tongue coat along with migraines, this prescription is the best choice.

Blood stasis headache

Typical manifestations: stubborn headache with fixed stabbing pain. The tongue will be dark or purplish and may have red or dark spots.

Treatment Principle: Promoting blood circulation to remove blood stasis.

Orifice-freeing Blood-Quickening Decoction (*Tōng Qiào Huó Xuě Tāng*) 通窍活血汤

Common Name	Pinyin	Chinese Name	Latin Name	Dose
Musk	*Shè xiāng*	麝香	Moschus	0.15g
Peach kernel	*Táo rén*	桃仁	Semen Persicae	9g
Carthamus flower	*Hóng huā*	红花	Flos Carthami	9g
Red peony root	*Chì sháo*	赤芍	Radix Paeoniae Rubra	3g
Chuanxiong rhizome	*Chuān xiōng*	川芎	Rhizoma Chuanxiong	3g
Scallion white	*Cōng bái*	葱白	Bulbus Allii Fistulosi	3 roots
Fresh ginger	*Shēng jiāng*	生姜	Rhizoma Zingiberis Recens	9g
Jujube fruit	*Dà zǎo*	大枣	Fructus Jujubae	7 fruits

This prescription was created by the famous Doctor Wang Qing-ren of the Qing Dynasty (1644 C.E. - 1911 C.E.), and is used to expel blood stasis. Recently, research has found this prescription is able to treat migraines due to blood stasis caused by vasospasms[38].

❹ Other forms of Chinese medicinals

Prepared medicines

Many practitioners today, especially those following Japanese or Taiwanese herbal methods, may also prescribe powdered herbs known as granules, pre-made tablets, capsules or syrups. This is probably the easiest way to take Chinese medicinals as it is similar to taking a biomedical pharmaceutical. The practitioner gives you the bottle (or bottles) of pills, tells you how many to take and how often, and when the time comes, you simply take the proper number of pills with warm water. The advantages over decoctions are obvious as you can avoid the cooking process and the strange taste. The major disadvantage may not be as obvious, but it is significant.

The reason Chinese medicine is so effective is that treatment can be tailored to exactly match the patient's individual pattern of disharmony. With Chinese medicinals, this is achieved by blending together a combination of substances that correspond to the presenting patterns. While formulas are helpful in that they serve as a guide to the treatment of the most common patterns, in almost all cases a formula will need to be modified to fit the patient exactly. The formula represented in a bottle of prepared medicine is unlikely to perfectly line up with a given patient's condition. Some parts of the patient's condition may remain unaddressed, and some parts of the formula may be inappropriate for the patient. This is why prepared medicines are usually used near the end of treatment, in order to "consolidate the treatment effect" by giving mild, long-term treatment directed at the patient's primary pattern. That being said, some practitioners combine two, three, or even more different prepared medicines to more accurately cover the patient's presentation.

There are total of six prepared medicines of plant origin that have been officially approved by the government for migraine use in China. They are:

❶ *Qī Yè Shén An Piàn* (Seven Leaves Spirit-Calming Pill)

This prepared medicine comes from plants containing protopanoxadiol. This substance can relieve pain, calm the nerves, and reduce inflammation. It can also nourish and adjust the central nervous system without adverse reactions

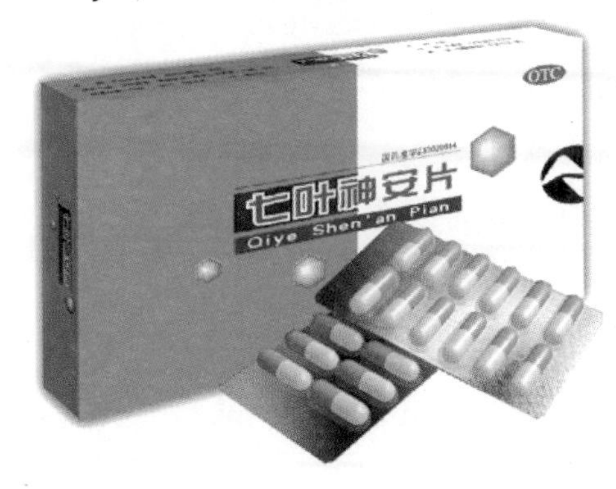

such as drowsiness, which is a very common side-effect of biomedical pain drugs.

Dosage: two pills three times / day. Two weeks is one course of treatment.

❷ ***Shén Qí Quán Tiān Má Jiāo Náng***
(Entirely marvelous gastrodia capsule)

This Chinese prepared medicine calms the liver to stop wind, relieve pain, eliminate convulsions, nourishes yin and blood, reinforces qi and essence, and calms the nerves. Dosage: two pills three times / day. Two weeks is one course of treatment.

❸ ***Fù Fāng Yáng Jiǎo Jiāo Náng***
(Complex goat horn prescription)

Promotes blood flow to expel wind and calms the liver to stop pain.

Dosage: five pills 3 times / day. Two weeks is one course of treatment.

❹ ***Yáng Xuě Qīng Nǎo Kē Lì***
(Blood-nourishing brain-clearing granules)

Nourishes blood and calms the liver, promotes blood circulation to remove channel obstructions and stops pain.

Dosage: one bag two times / day. Two weeks is one course of treatment.

❺ ***Nǎo An Piàn***
(Brain-calming pill)

This product can promote blood flow to expel stagnant blood, reinforce qi, smooth the channels, and stop pain.

Dosage: one pill, two-three times / day. Three weeks is one course of treatment.

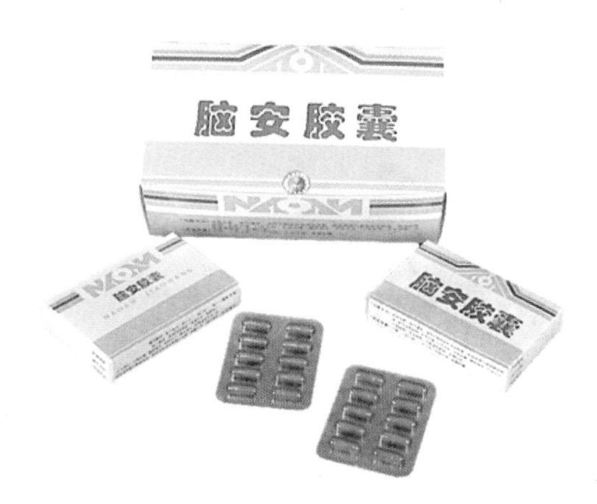

❻ ***Tài Jí Tōng Tiān Yè***
(Absolute celestial connection liquid)

Promotes blood flow to expel stagnant blood, smooth qi flow in the channels, expels wind to stop pain.

Dosage: 10 ml two-three times / day. Seven days is one course of treatment.

These formulas contain many different combinations of medicinals, but since they are all designed specifically for migraine patients, they have much in common. Since the most common symptom in a migraine headache patient is pain, every one of these products contains medicinals that can stop pain. Also, since internal blood stasis, qi stagnation, and qi deficiency are also common, many of these patterns are addressed. Since each product is slightly different, a trained professional will need to help you choose the best one.

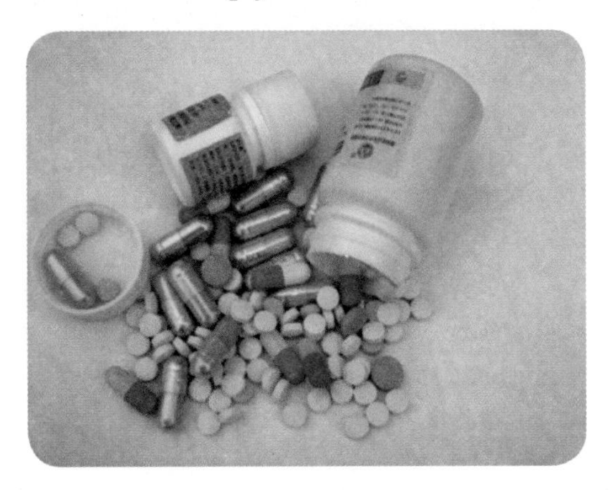

Granules

Chinese medicinals in granule form is a modern creation and represents a middle path between decoctions and prepared medicines. To make granules, individual herbs or whole formulas are cooked down until a concentrated powder remains. These are packaged and can be combined to fit the patient's exact pattern. The patient takes the granule packets, empties one into a cup or container, pours hot water over the mixture, stirs to dissolve, and drinks. This allows for a more convenient preparation along with individualized formula design. However, it is generally thought that taking Chinese medicinals in granule form is slightly less effective than decoctions. Despite this, granules have become popular with many patients and practitioners in recent years due to their ease of preparation.

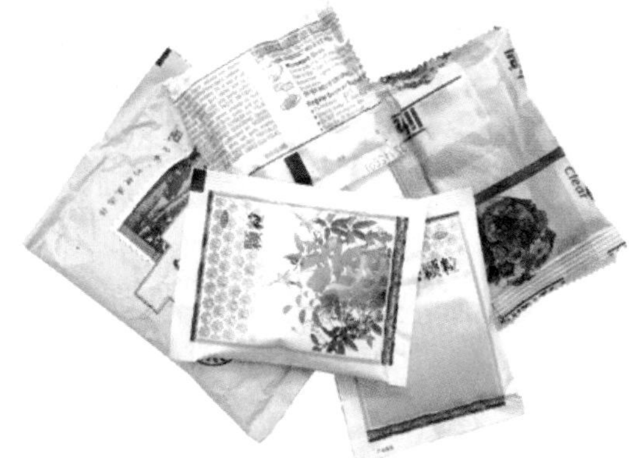

External application

Chinese medicinals are sometimes prepared so that they may be applied directly to the skin to be absorbed superficially. External applications are usually used for problems of the skin and superficial channels. They are used often in dermatology, but are also often used to treat pain, numbness, and injury of a local area. Patients with migraine headaches may be given a formula to use externally in order to treat pain.

The simplest way to make an external application is to boil herbs like you would a decoction and use the warm liquid as a wash. External applications do not need to be as specific as decoctions that are taken internally. For this reason, prepared products in oil, cream, or tincture form are often given. This form of treatment allows for more direct application of medicinals to the area where there is a problem and bypasses the digestive tract, avoiding possible problems in digestion.

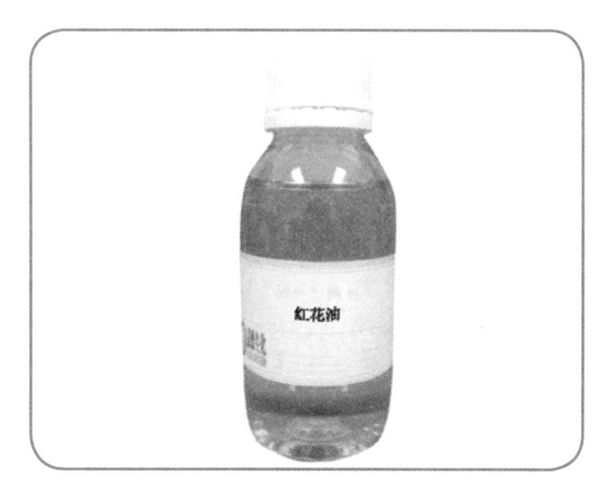

Attention!

The information in this section is not meant to be a cookbook for you to choose from. It is presented in order to help you understand more about Chinese medicine. The selection of medicinals must be done by a trained practitioner.

3. Translated Research

❶A clinical study in Shandong University of Chinese Medicine in 2006 observed effects of *Xiaoyao Nose Drops* (XYND) in stopping episodes of migraine headaches. This was a randomized double blind placebo-controlled study, with 126 patients evenly assigned to two groups. The treatment group was given XYND and the control group received a placebo, over 30 days. The total effective rate and the effect in alleviating acute headaches was observed. Before and after treatment, blood flow in various parts of the brain was measured. Results showed a headache alleviating rate of 93% in the treatment group, while the rate in the control group was only 20%. Blood viscosity, plasma viscosity and fibrinogen lowered significantly in the treatment group in comparison to before treatment or in the control group after treatment. The velocity of blood flow in all cerebral arteries also lowered significantly in the treatment group, also showing significant difference in comparison with before treatment or with the control group after treatment. So, XYND is effective in alleviating migraine headaches, and worth applying in clinical practice[39].

❷ An experimental study in Shandong University of Chinese Medicine in 2002 observed the treatment of migraines using the formula *Shu Tian Ning Granule* (STNG). The study involved 90 patients with migraines divided into three groups: the treated group was given STNG 9g, three times a day; the control Group A was treated with another prepared Chinese medicinal pill, *Yang Jiao Capsule*, 5 capsules, three times a day; and control Group B treated with flunarizine hydrochloride capsule, 5 mg once per day. The study lasted 28 days to observe the degree, length and frequency of pain attacks. The results showed that in the treated group, the marked effective rate was 57% and 90% of patients experienced some effect, a significant difference in comparison with control Group B, but with no difference in comparison with control Group A. In conclusion, STNG could improve cerebrovascular function and ease vascular tension in patients with migraines[40].

❸ A study in Beijing and Hebei, China, in 2007 among a group of 46 patients with migraine headaches showed that the curative effect of *Quan Tian Ma Capsule* to treat migraine headaches was quite promising even though the patients came from different ages and different family histories[41].

❹ A study in Zhejiang, China in 2007 among a group of 36 patients with migraine headaches showed that the curative effect by using *San Chong Ding Tong Decoction* to treat migraine headaches was visible[42]. The formula was modified according each individual's pattern. The overall curative effect was excellent.

❺ A study in Jiangsu, China in 2007 among a group of 38 patients with migraine headaches showed that the curative effect by using *Modified Chai Hu Long Gu Mu Li Decoction* was satisfactory[43].

❻ A study in Hebei, China in 2007 among a group of 105 patients with migraine headaches showed that the method of clearing heat, calming the liver and eliminating wind to stop pain was effective in cases where no biomedical treatment had been effective[44].

❼ A study in Beijing, China in 2007 compared patients treated with *Man Jing Zi Tou Feng Decoction* to patients that had received Ligustrazine Hydrochloride Injection to relieve migraines and showed that the results of *Man Jing Zi Tou Feng Decoction* were satisfactory in comparison[45].

Tui Na – Massage

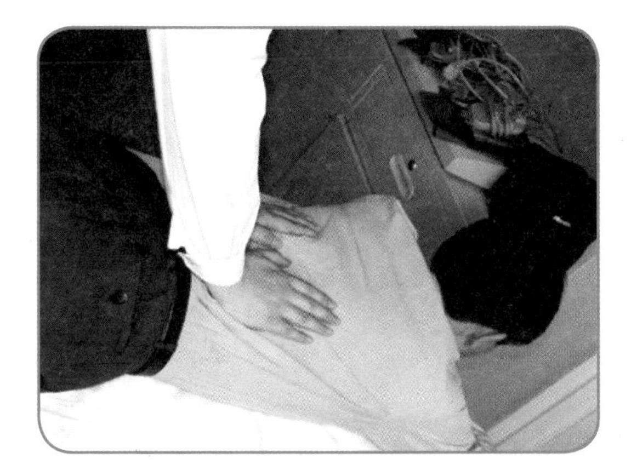

1. What Is Tui Na?

Tui na, literally "pushing and grasping", but better translated as massage, is a manual practice of manipulating the body performed by highly-skilled practitioners. By stimulating the acupuncture points and channels with well-honed techniques, the channels can be opened and the flow of qi and blood will be promoted and regulated. The body's qi will be strengthened and so will its resistance to disease. Tui na is an important element of Chinese medicine and is popular with everyday people as it is simple, convenient, effective, and inexpensive.

Tui na is irreplaceable as a natural kind of physical therapy. You may have already tried other kinds of massage, but the tui na of Chinese medicine is unique because it is deeply rooted in Chinese medical theory. For example, according to the theory of Chinese medicine, pain is either due to stagnation or deficiency, with local stagnation of the flow of qi and blood being the most common cause. Tui na can relieve this kind of pain by applying forceful, regular, smooth, and penetrating manipulations in order to remove stagnation and promote the flow of qi and blood. Pain with a different diagnosis would be treated differently, in accordance to theory. As in all aspects of Chinese medicine, applying individualized treatment is of primary importance. Discovering the unique pattern of disharmony in each patient is vital in order to apply the correct treatment methods.

In the treatment of migraines, tui na is effective, though it often plays a supplementary role. Manual stimulus on acupuncture points (acupressure) will also produce effects similar to acupuncture according to the theory of Chinese medicine. Tui na is convenient and also may sound safer to those fearful of needles. What's more important is that it is at least as effective as needles. You will be relaxed and refreshed every time you leave the clinic.

2. Treatment Methods

1 Point Selection

According to channels

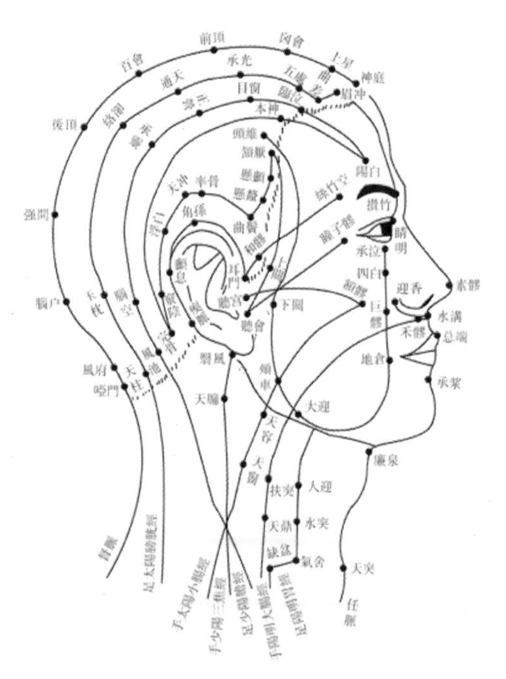

This method includes selecting points both near to and far from the pain site on channels that traverse the area of pain. Points near the pain are on the head and face, such as EX-HN3 (*yìn táng*), EX-HN5 (*tài yáng*), DU 20 (*bǎi huì*), GB 20 (*fēng chí*), etc. Points far from the pain are found on the four limbs, such as LI 4 (*hé gǔ*) and LI 11 (*qū chí*) on the large intestine channel, ST 36 (*zú sān li*) on the stomach channel, LV 2 (*xíng jiān*) on the liver channel, etc. The channels these points lie on traverse different parts of the head and face.

According to pain location

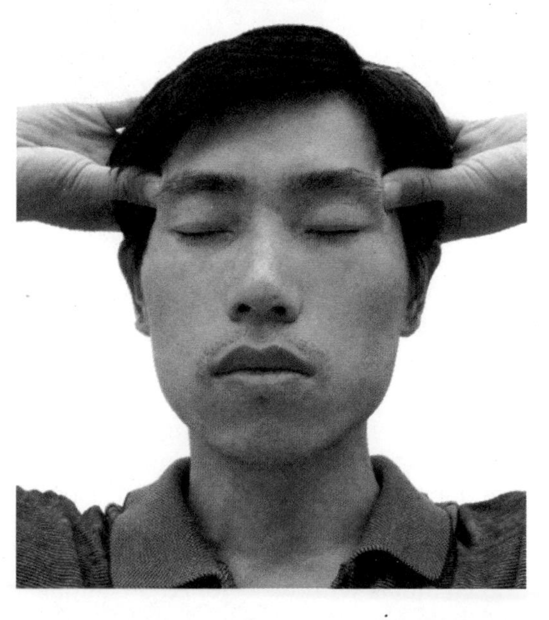

Pressure points of the head are located wherever the headache is focused. The intention is to eliminate symptoms by relieving tension or spasms of local blood vessels, nerves and muscle tissue.

Generally, both of the above methods will be used simultaneously.

2 Manipulation techniques

Though manipulation techniques are learned on their own, they are almost always used in combination with several other techniques.

Pressing is the application of force against to part of the body or acupuncture points.

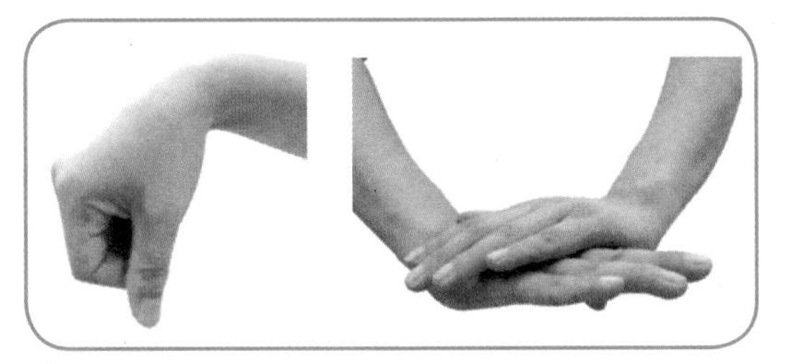

Pointing uses the top of the knuckles to press certain acupuncture points. It is done with the hands in a fist.

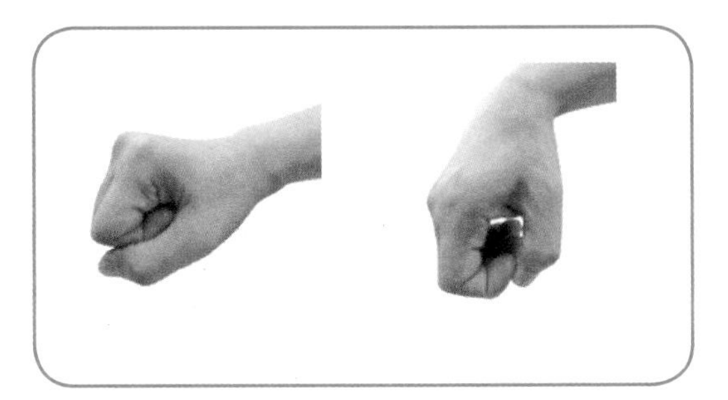

Rubbing reduction uses the or base of the palm to press into the region, then rotate softly to spur circulation.

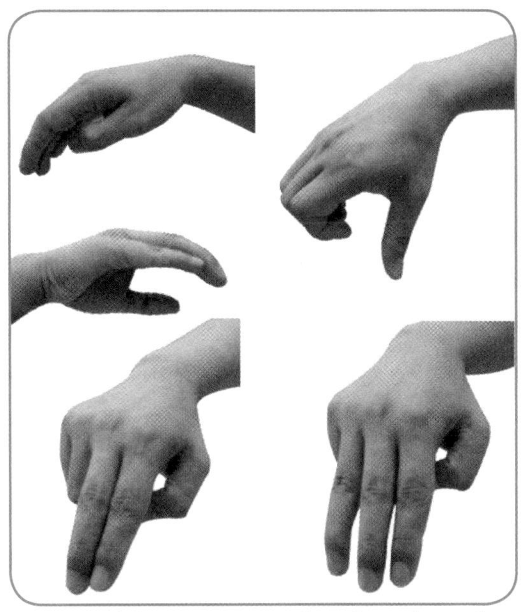

Pushing presses the thumb, palm, or other part of the body firmly into the acupuncture point or part of the patient's body, while roaming linearly or in curves along the muscle.

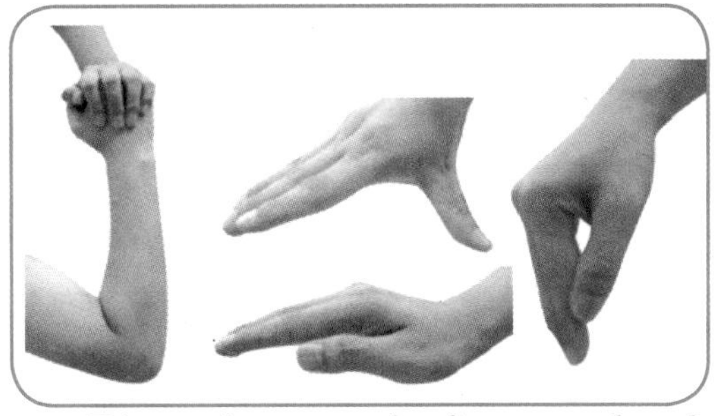

Dispersing uses the fingers to brush the temporal part of the head back and forth.

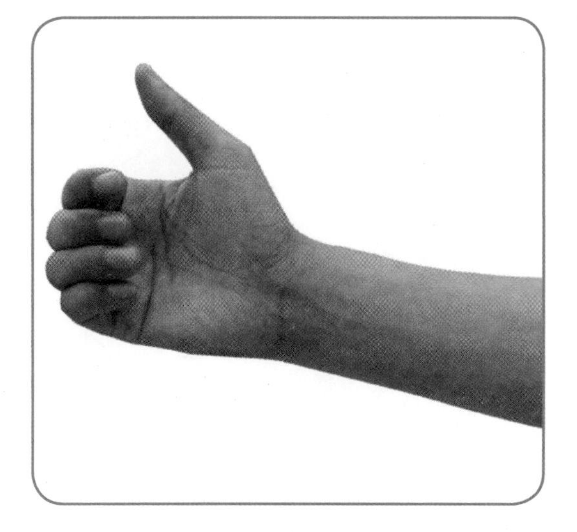

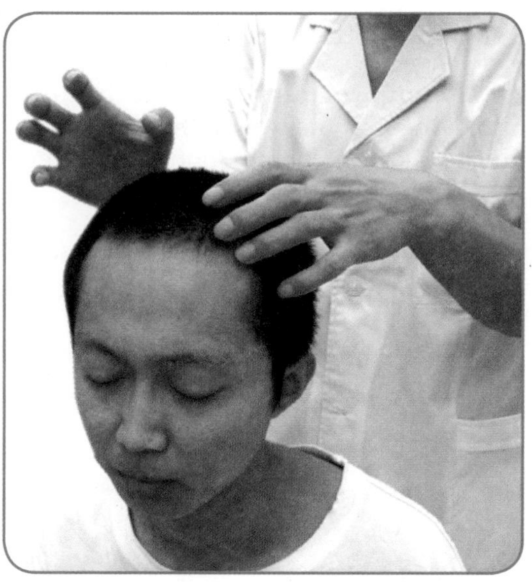

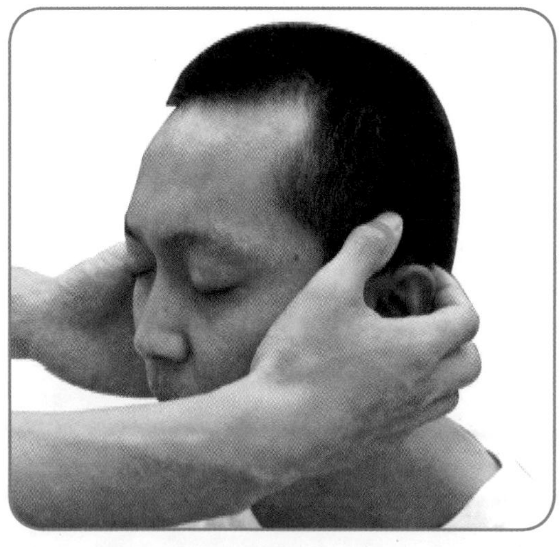

Pecking uses the five fingers slightly bent and separated in a relaxed position. The wrist joint is flexed and extended to tap acupuncture points swiftly and rhythmically just as chickens peck rice.

3. What Will Treatment Be Like?

After inquiring about your condition and performing a detailed examination, the practitioner will decide on a tui na procedure based on the pattern identification. Since tui na is a direct, manual therapy, treatment can take place almost anywhere and in many positions, but most often patients will be asked to lie on their back or stomach. Sometimes the massage will be done in the sitting position. If necessary, the position may be changed during the treatment.

A pair of trained hands is all that is necessary for a tui na treatment to be per-

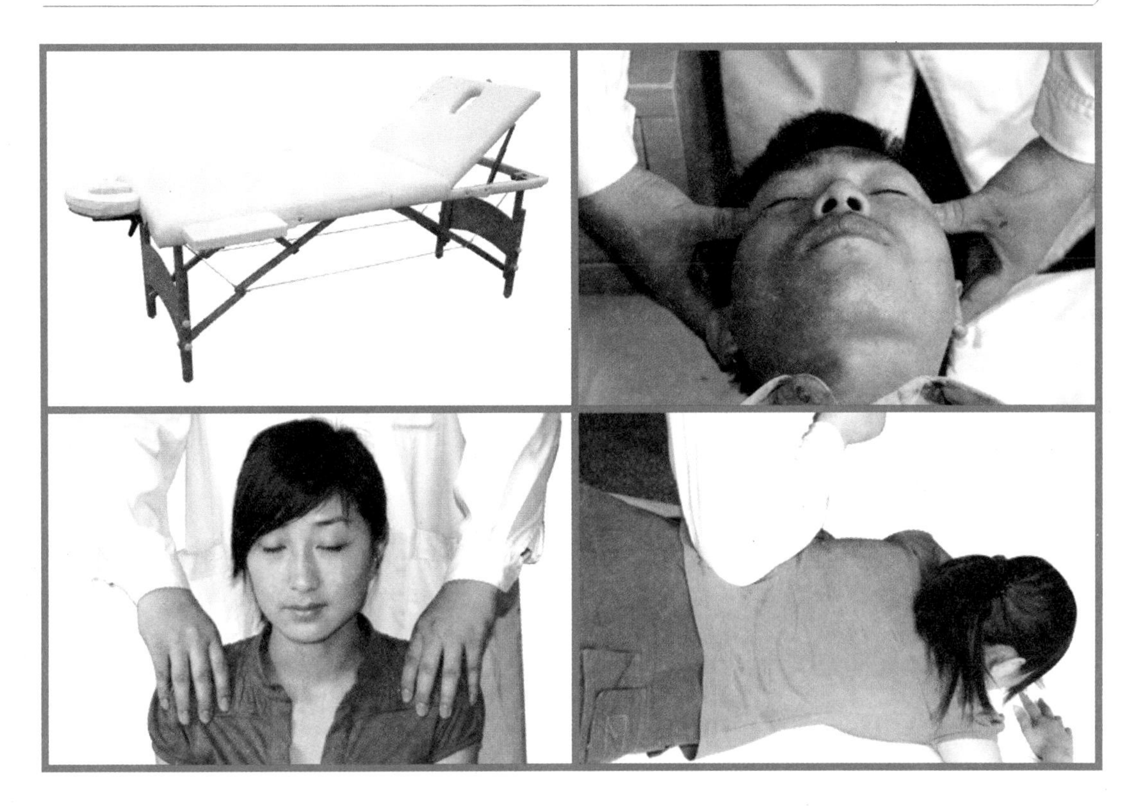

formed. That's why the manipulations are called *"shǒu fǎ"* (techniques of the hands) in Chinese. Other parts of the practitioner's body might also be used, such as elbows and arms. Occasionally, a practitioner might use some kind of massage tools.

Special oil or medicinal paste may sometimes be used to lubricate and protect the skin and for their own therapeutic effects. The most common ingredients are common oily substances like lanolin or beeswax mixed with medicinals that invigorate qi and blood. Sometimes medicinal pastes are specially made to treat certain conditions. For example, one kind of paste for deficiency pain, another for stagnation pain; one kind for the upper body and a different type for the lower half.

Techniques of manipulation and point selection will be made on the basis of the patient's condition and existing patterns. Since the fundamental pathomechanism of migraine headaches in Chinese medicine is qi and blood stasis, points and techniques that promote the circulation of qi and blood will usually be part of the

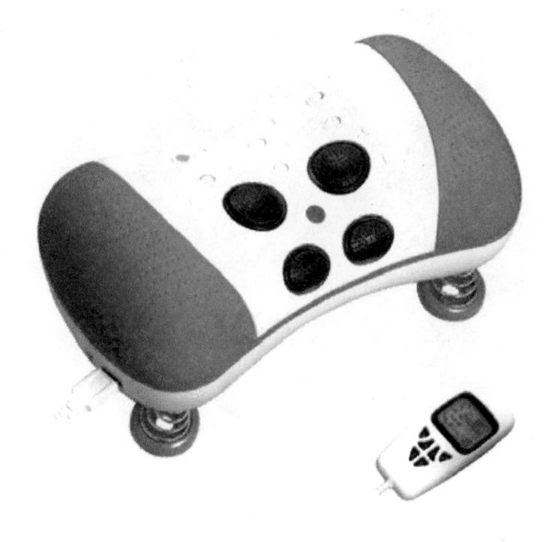

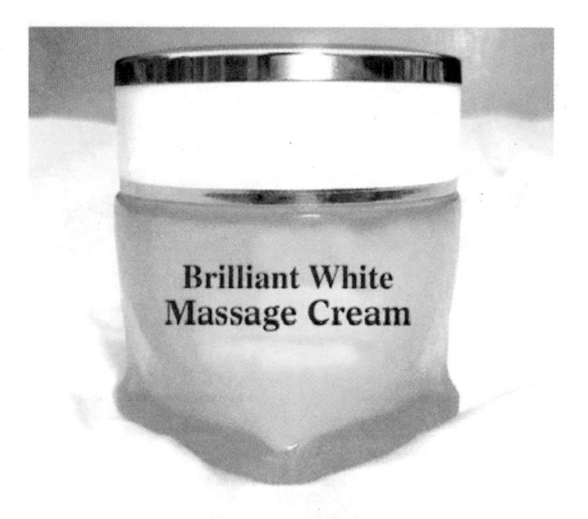

treatment. Other points will be chosen according to the patient's pattern diagnosis or symptoms.

4. At-home Massage

Tui na is not as simple as it looks, even though many of the procedures look like actions performed every day such as pushing, grasping, pressing and kneading. It is actually a set of highly-skilled techniques and expert movements that are performed according to Chinese medical theory. It is targeted at the system of channels and acupuncture points throughout the body. Therefore, the manipulations must be performed by trained practitioners to promote internal self-adjustment of the channel system without harming the local tissues of the body. The effect of tui na depends more on the skill with which the manipulations are performed rather than on the sheer force of the pressure. Force, even a small amount, applied improperly can be harmful to the body. It is not suggested to perform or receive tui na treatments that you have observed in the clinic on or by your friends or family members without the presence of an instructor.

Nonetheless, there are some self-massage practices which are safe, simple, convenient, and designed for migraine patients to exercise their body and mind and serve as a supplement to the management of headaches.

There are many different manipulations in tui na, and hundreds of acupuncture points and body parts these techniques can be used on. To make things

simple, we have chosen some routines that can be performed on the patient by a friend or family member, or that can be performed by the patient alone. Please note that there are numerous tui na routines and self-massage protocols recommended for migraine patients. We have tried to choose a few that have some evidence of their effectiveness, but routines learned from your practitioner or other sources may work as well. The most important thing is to find something that helps you and feels good.

❶ Head and face massage

This routine is performed while sitting down. The person receiving the massage should sit upright with a straight back. Stabilize the emotions, concentrate the mind. The masseuse begins by rubbing their hands together warmly, and places one on each EX-HN5 (*tài yáng*). Then massage the point 10 - 20 times clockwise and 10 - 20 times counterclockwise.

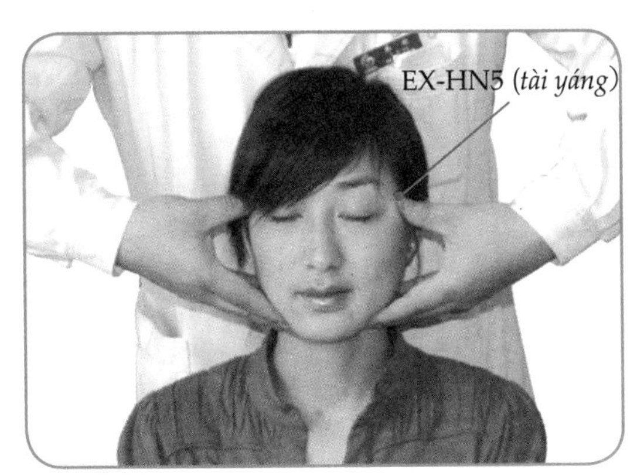

Step 1: Begin by spreading 18 times from the center of the eyebrow to the hairline with the lateral surface of the two thumbs. Then, spread 9 times from the middle of the eyebrows EX-HN3 (yìn táng) to EX-HN5 (*tài yáng*) with the pad of the thumbs.

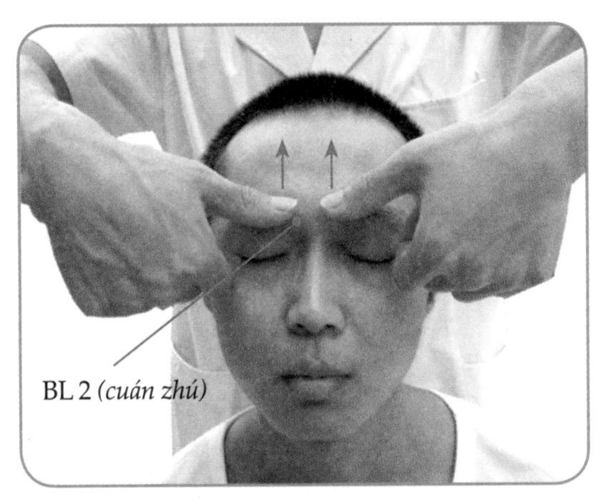

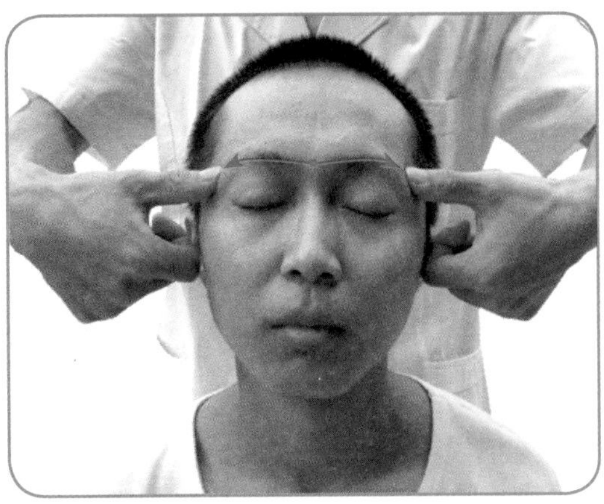

Step 2: Rub 9 times from in front of the ears to EX-HN5 (*tài yáng*) with the two forefingers and middle fingers. The forefinger and middle finger push towards the point and then back towards the starting point in front of the ear.

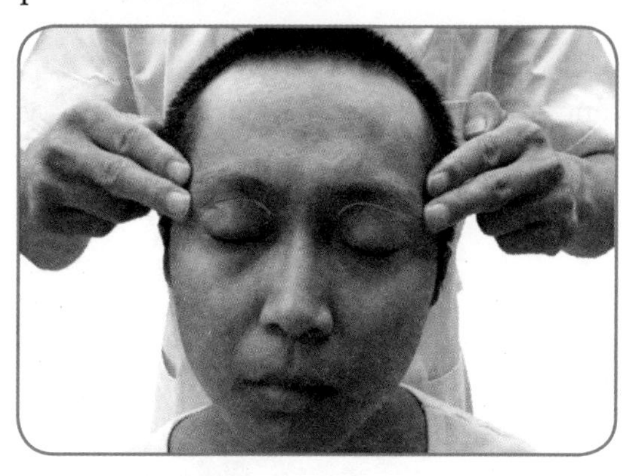

Step 3: Push with the thumb tips 7 - 9 times from inner corner of the eyes to the outer corner of the eyes along the bony ridge that surrounds the eyes. Then, place the two thumbs on EX-HN5 (*tài yáng*), and lightly spread outward from the eye sockets 9 times.

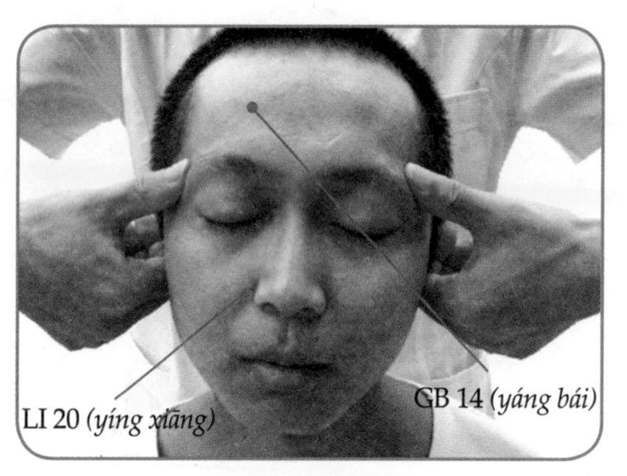

Step 4: Press and knead both EX-HN5 (*tài yáng*) with the thumbs clockwise and counterclockwise 9 times, and press BL 2 (*cuán zhú*), EX-HN4 (*yú yāo*), GB 14 (*yáng bái*), ST 2 (*sì bái*), and LI 20 (*yíng xiāng*) for 15 seconds each. Each point exists on both the right and left side of the head. Both should be pressed. Then press DU 20 (*bǎi huì*) at the top of the head with the two forefingers or middle fingers for 2 minutes.

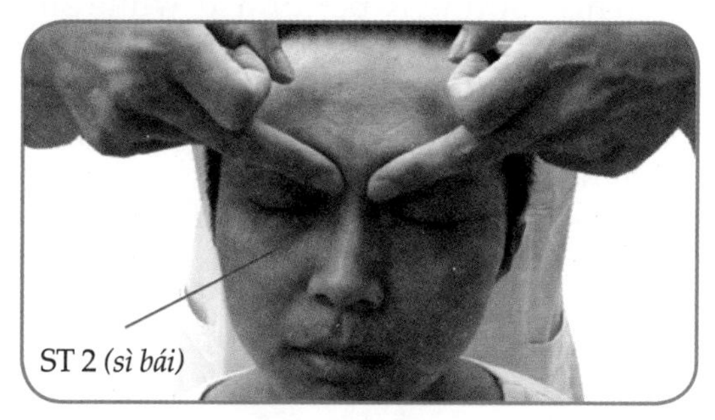

Step 5: Put one hand on one side of head for support. With five fingers of the other hand spread apart and bent slightly, use the fingers to push and scrape back and forth beside the temporal bone. Next, switch to the other hand. Push and scrape 18 times per side.

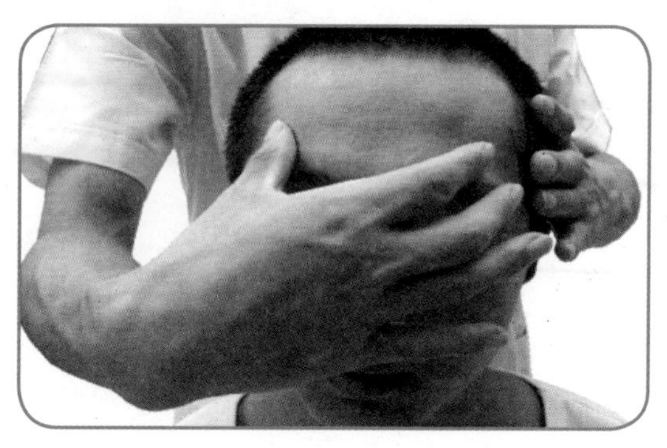

Step 6: Knead 49 times at EX-HN3 (*yìn táng*), and using the thumbs spread outwards towards the ears.

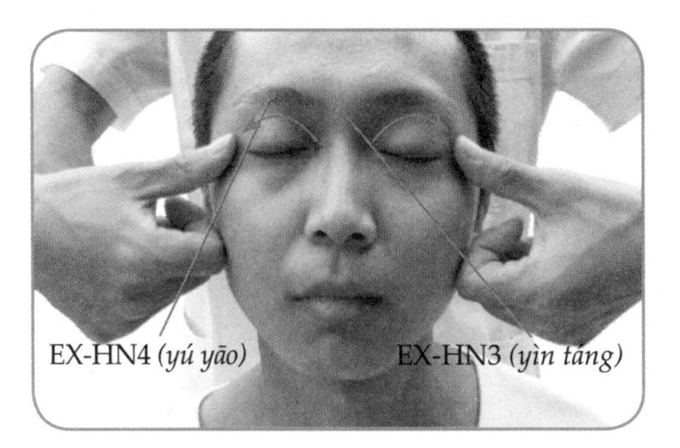

❷ Neck and nape massage

This routine is performed while sitting down.

Step 1: Locate the point *qiáo gōng* on the neck. Push and swab both points on each side of the neck with the thumbs 9 times each. Only do one side at a time to avoid choking the patient or causing a cough.

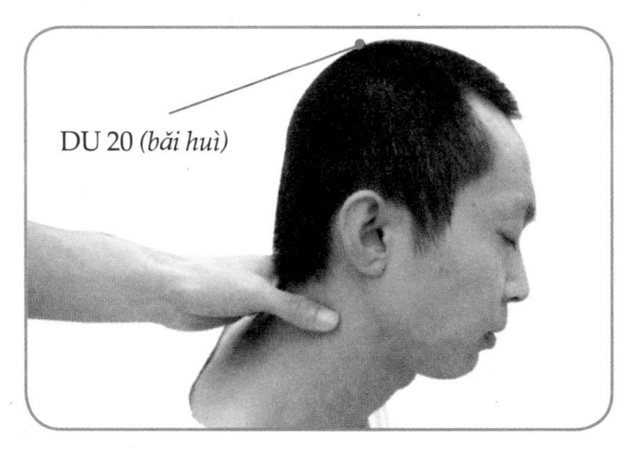

Step 2: With all five fingers separated and bent slightly, press from the forehead to the crown of the head. Next press both sides of the head just above the ears 3 times back and forth.

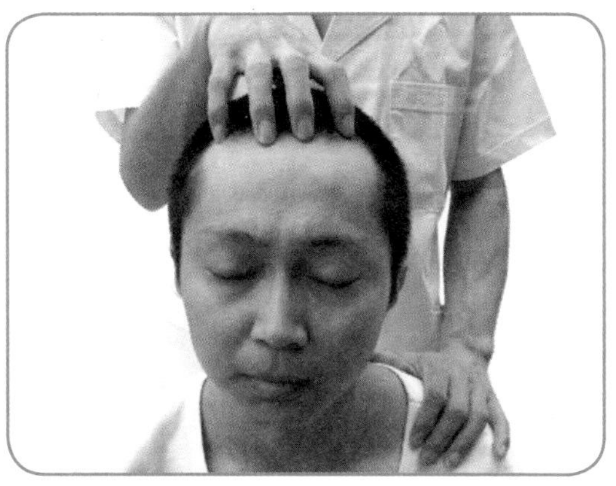

Step 3: Grasp and pinch the two side muscles of the neck from top to bottom 7 times.

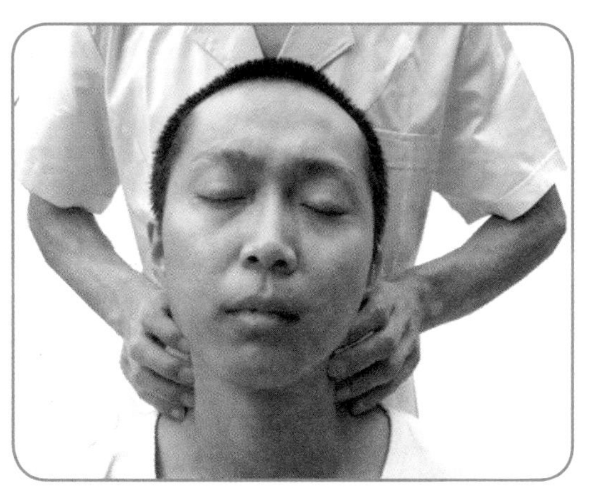

Step 4: Press and knead GB 20 (*fēng chí*) with the thumbs clockwise and counterclockwise 9 times each way.

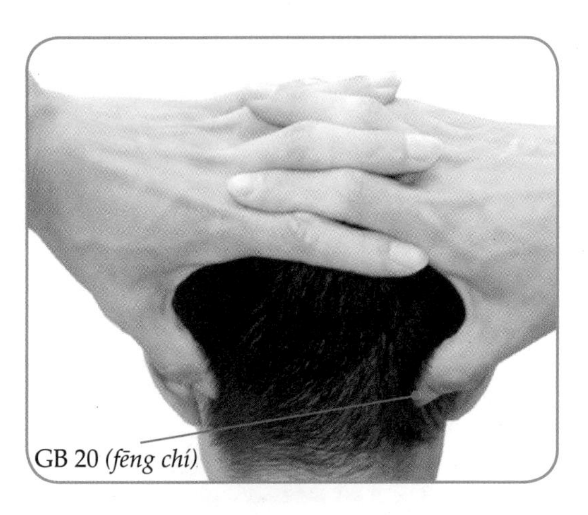

Step 5: One hand supports the neck, while the other hand claps DU 20 (*bǎi huì*) lightly. Repeat with each hand 10 times.

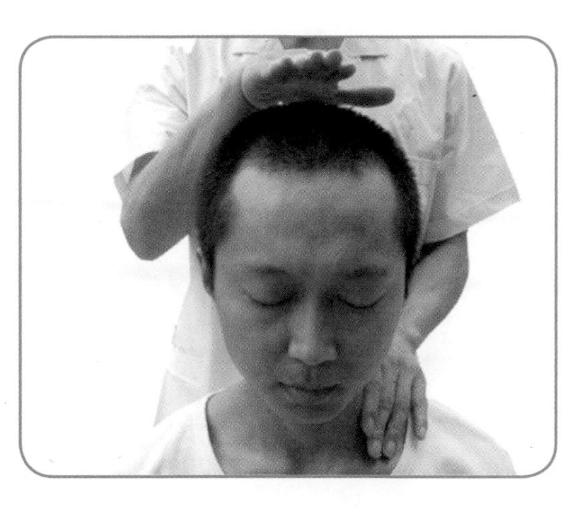

Step 6: Both hands comb the hair and shake the ears 9 times. Afterwards, relax, sit silently and regulate the breath for 3 minutes.

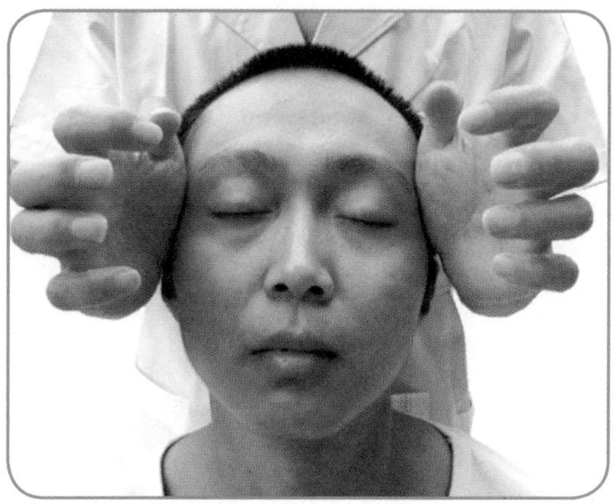

❸ Contraindications for tui na

- Serious underlying diseases, such as heart, brain or lung diseases
- Infectious diseases like hepatitis, tuberculosis, erysipelas, or osteomyelitis
- Malignant tumors, though other areas may be massaged
- Hematological diseases with a tendency to heavy bleeding
- Bone fractures, though other areas may be massaged

- Diseased skin areas, though other areas may be massaged

- Especially weak condition, drunk, very hungry, or full

- Over the abdominal and sacral regions during pregnancy

5. Translated Research

❶ Massage and Daoyin, 2003 relays a clinical study in which 50 cases of migraine were treated successfully using tui na. The cause of migraine in these cases was unkown, MRI and CT found nothing wrong in this patient population. Though these patients had been treated with biomedicine, none of them had been cured. In this study, massage relieved the symptoms without any internal treatment or medication[46].

❷ In 2003 Wang Zhen reported a case of magraine cured by massage. This case was first treated with pharmaceutical medication, but frequently relapsed after only a few days. By massage, the patient finally recovered[47].

❸ Also in 2003, Wen Bo Ping, Meng Hai Bin and Chen Lin studied the massage treatment of migraines of cervical origin that had previously been discussed in medical journals. They found that massage given according to anatomical considerations is a relatively effective method. The clinical application is quite successful[48].

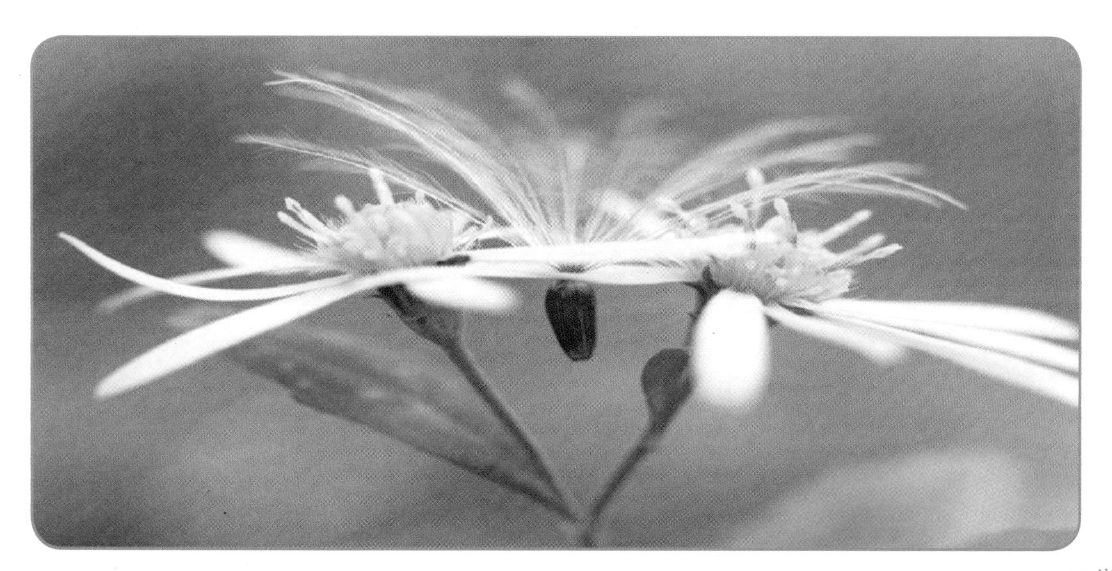

At-home Therapies

Apart from the treatment methods mentioned above, a simple hand, ear, and foot massage can be done at home with the guidance of a practitioner. The routine below is based on the holistic view of Chinese medicine, together with channel theory and modern holographic theory. Holographic therapies on the hands and feet are commonly known as reflexology.

Basic theory of reflexology

- There are reflex points (or areas) on various holographic units in the body, such as the feet, hands, ears, etc.

- If the function of an organ in the body becomes abnormal, there will also be tenderness that can be detected on the corresponding reflex area.

- In turn, stimulating a reflex point can help to adjust the function of the related organ and the body as a whole can be returned to balance.

By stimulating the reflex points on the hands, ears, or feet, the internal organs can be stimulated and regulated. So by stimulating the brain area of the ear, for instance, your brain may be activated. You can do this routine at home by yourself or with the help of a friend or family member.

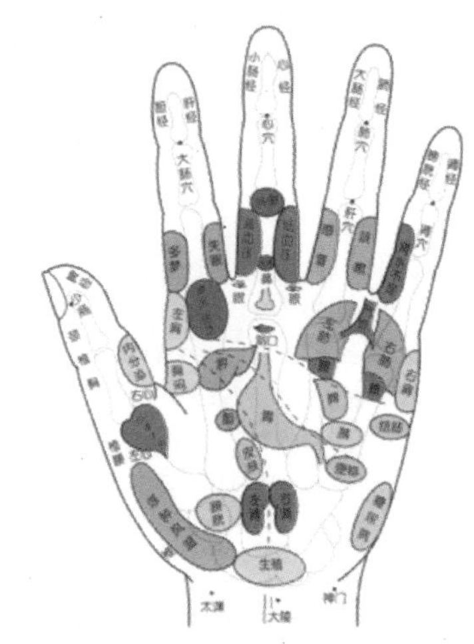

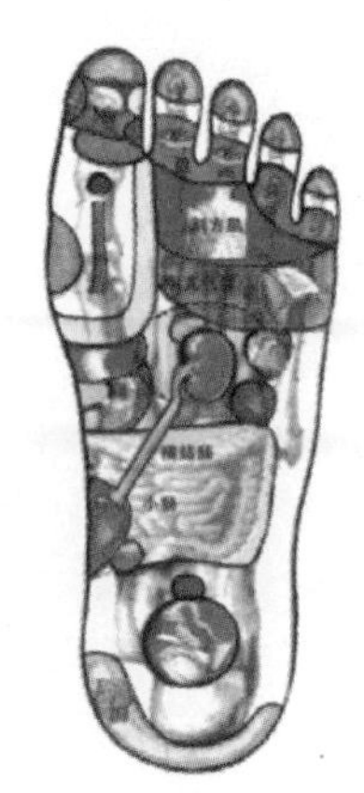

Hand, ear, and foot self-massage

Gentle self-massage of the hands, ears, and feet can be done by people of all ages and conditions. With just a five to ten minute massage you can feel relaxed and relieved. You can follow the procedure recommended here, or that recommended by your practitioner.

Wash your hands, face, and feet with warm water. Play a light music if you like. Sit comfortably. Relax yourself and empty your mind. You can also use lotion if your skin is dry.

- Rub your hands gently as if you are washing them.

- Stretch the palm of your hand with the other one, gently pressing the palm and stretching the muscles of the hand.

- Press the reflexology points shown on the illustration.

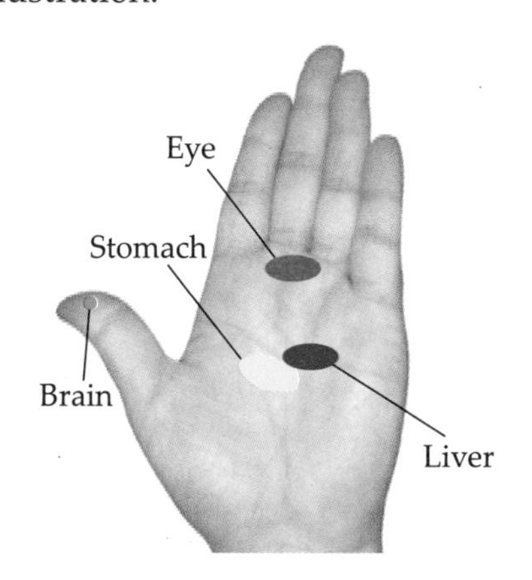

- Massage the muscles and tendons between the bones of the hand.

- Use your wrist to massage the opposite palm.

- Massage each finger and pull the fingers visualizing tension pouring out of the fingertips.

- Massage your face with your finger tips from jaw to cheeks using gentle, circular motions.

- Massage your ears all over and warm them with your hands.

- Stretch the lobes gently and press the points shown on the image.

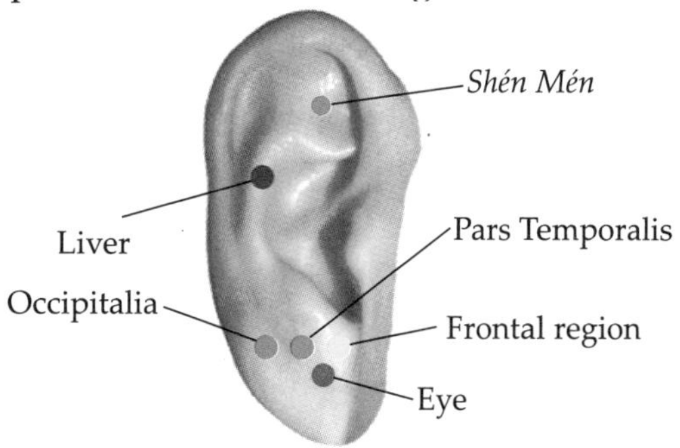

- Prop one foot in your lap and let the other rest extended in front of you.

- Massage one foot and when finished, change position and do the other.

- Put one hand on top of the foot and the other closer to your toes, then stroke from the toes to the ankle.

- Place your hands on the sole of the foot and massage the reflexology points shown in the image.

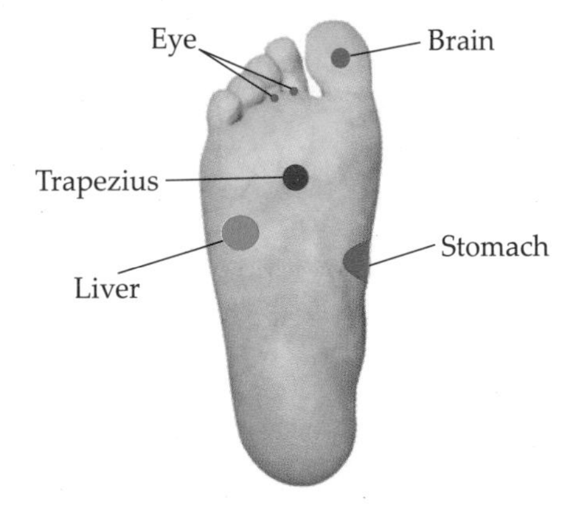

- Massage the whole foot and pull the toes visualizing the tension pulling out from the tip of toes.

- Press the arch of the foot with your wrist.

- Again put one hand on top of the foot and the other closer to your toes, then stroke from the toes to the ankle.

The above routine can be done every other day or twice a week. In a month you will feel better. Continue to massage yourself regularly to ensure a lasting effect.

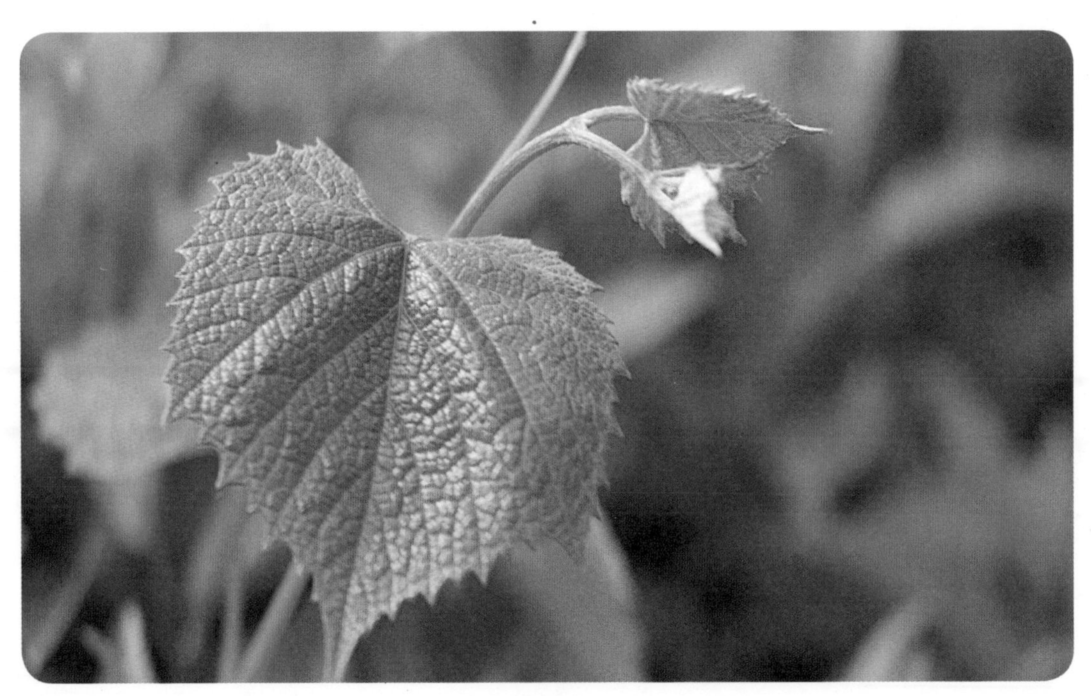

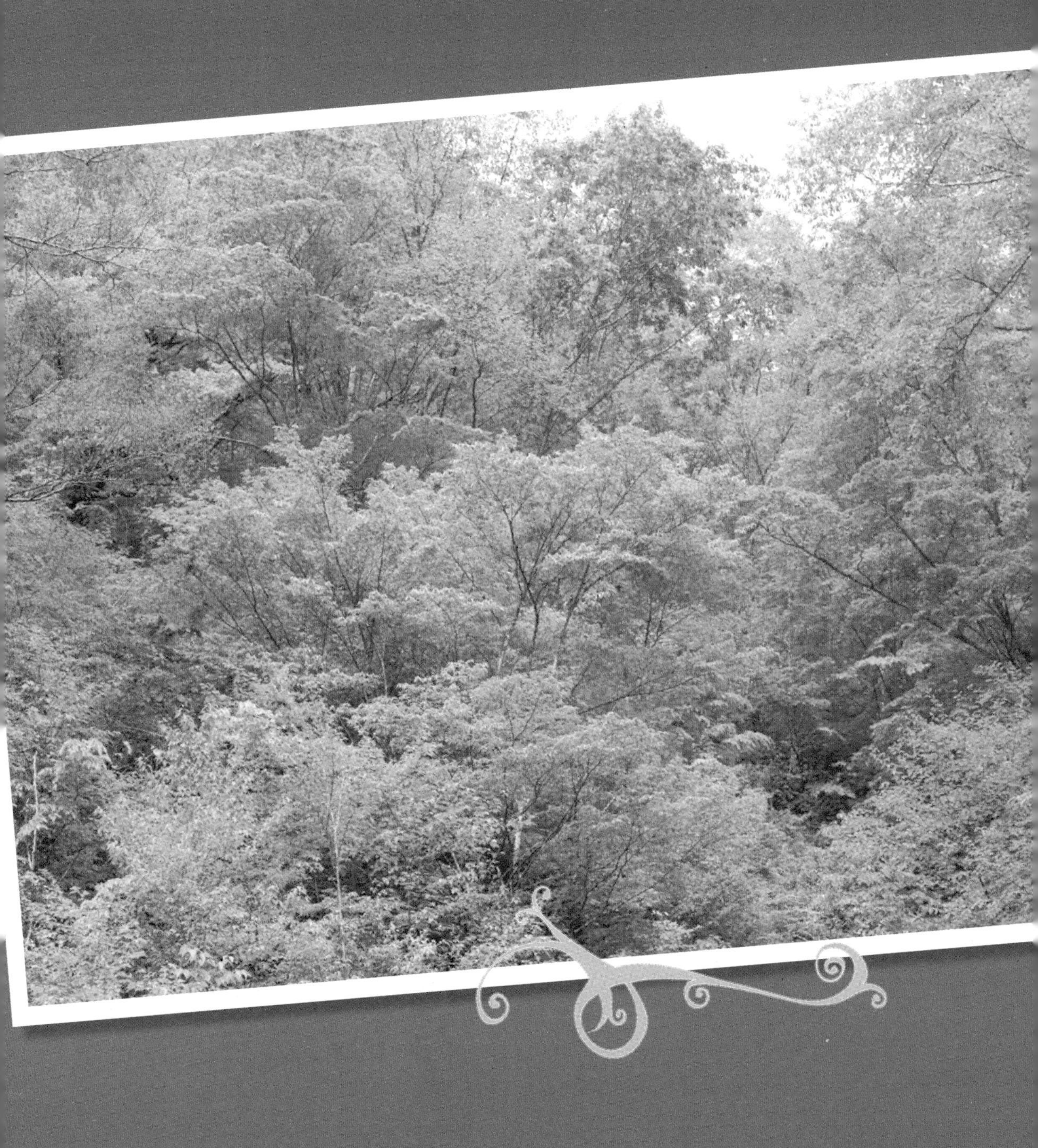

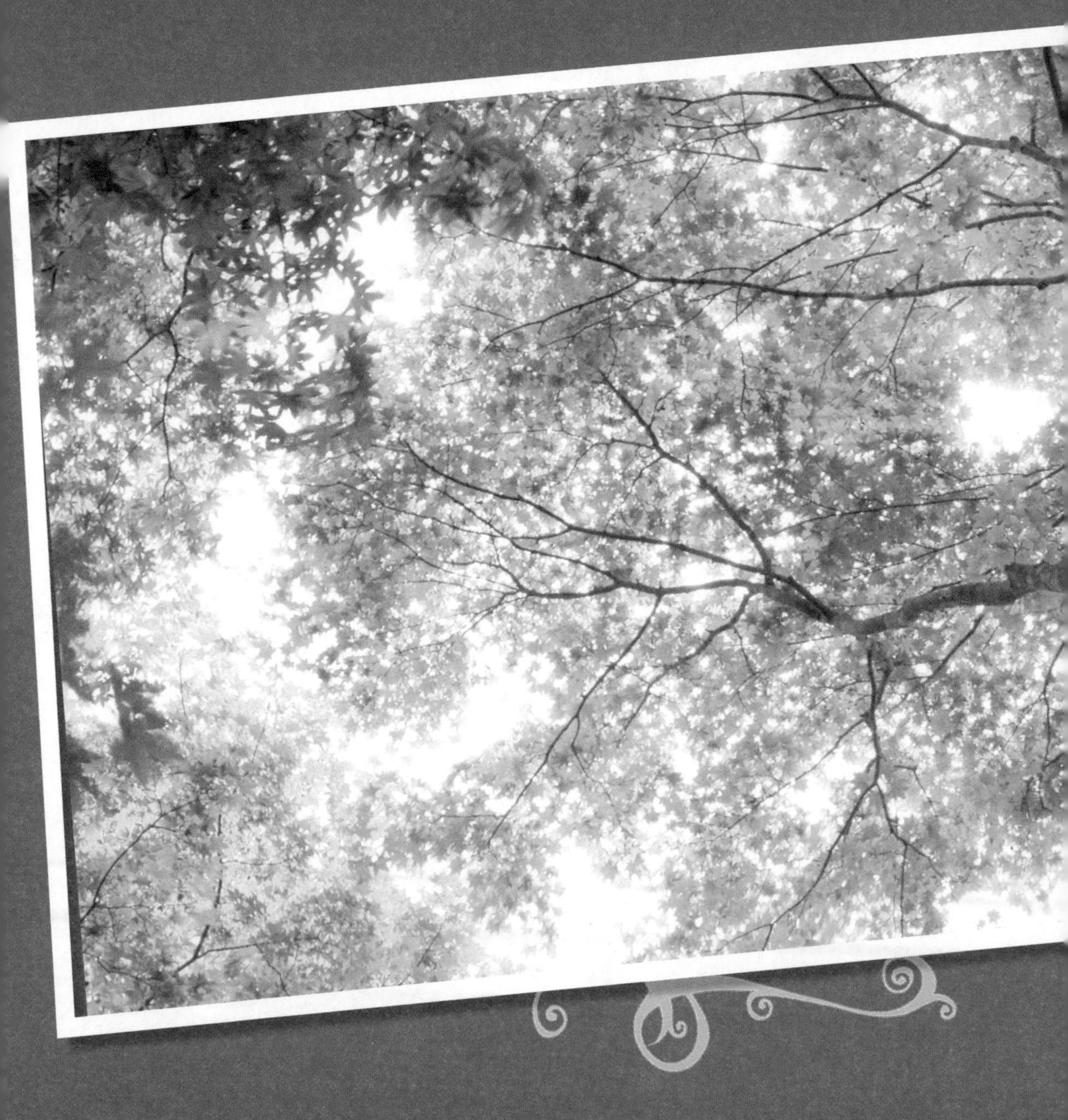

Chapter 5

Case Histories

This final chapter includes various case histories from real patients with migraine headaches. They represent the standard of care for migraine patients with Chinese medicine. As you have seen above, migraines have been rigorously studied both in the clinic and the laboratory. These cases are included to show you that by using this knowledge, real people have been able to bring their disease under control and lead healthy lives. You may notice that nearly all the histories involve treatment with herbal medicine, usually prescribed to be taken as a decoction every day for a number of weeks or months. For those who were initially attracted to treatment with Chinese medicine because of what they heard about acupuncture, we encourage you to give herbal medicine a fair trial. It is the most effective, safest, and fastest way to health with Chinese medicine. From reading this book, you will be able to understand something about the Chinese medical theory and treatment protocols.

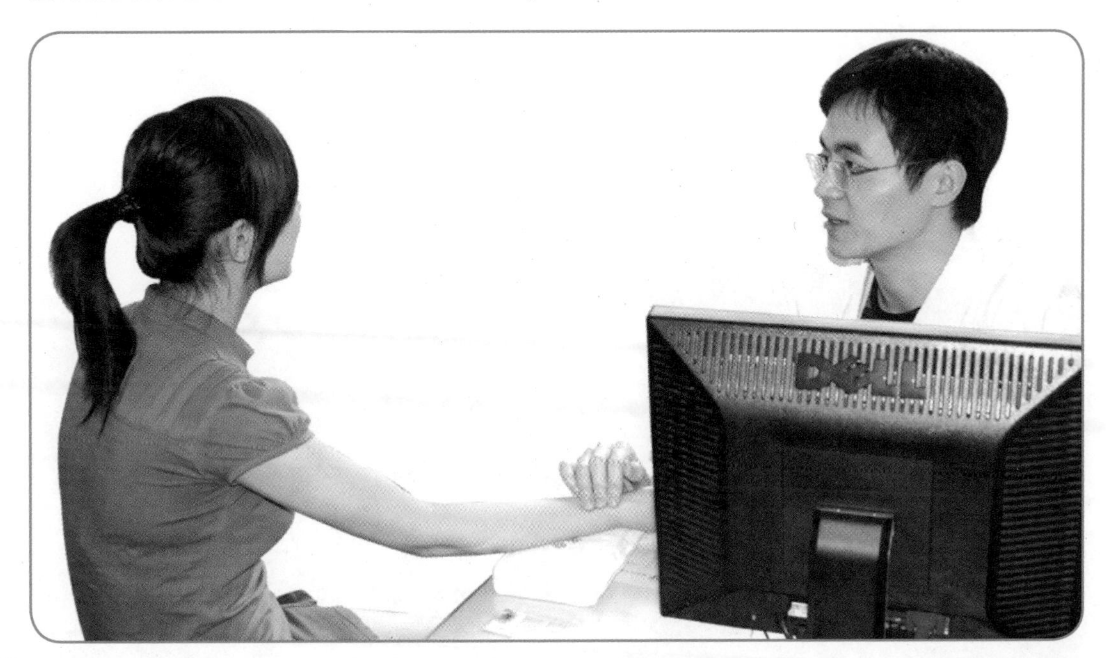

Case 1 - Migraine due to phlegm heat

Mrs. Chai is a 54 year old female who has had migraines for more than 30 years. Her first visit to the clinic was July 4, 1999. At this time, she was experiencing a headache about once per month, which lasted several days. After the attack, it was as though nothing had happened, everything returned to normal. No previous treatment had been successful.

During examination, it was determined the patient had blood stagnation due to the long duration of attacks. The strategy, therefore, was to move qi and blood. After treatment, her headaches still occurred as before. So, on the return visit the case was looked at more carefully. Her symptoms included a heavy feeling like her head was wrapped tightly, left eye socket that felt distended, stomach cramps with nausea, and a thick, greasy and slightly yellow coating on her tongue. The above symptoms indicated her headaches were due to a flaring up of phlegm heat, so the treatment method was changed to eliminate phlegm, descend turbidity, and clear heat. A medicinal formula that included tangerine peel, pinellia, chuanxiong, licorice, and other substances was given. Mrs. Chai took one dose per day, decocted with water.

After six doses, her symptoms were relieved, though she still had a bitter taste in her mouth. She was given a similar formula, but slightly modified to clear more heat. After three doses, all headache symptoms disappeared, but she still felt some stomach cramps and liked to lie down often. Again the above formula was used, but modified to regulate the digestion and stop the production of phlegm. After this last course of treatment Mrs. Chai experienced no further recurrence of headaches.

Case 2 - Migraine due to blood stasis

Mr. Chen was 38 years old. His first visit to the clinic was in April 1998. He had a head injury 20 years prior, after which his migraines began. Initially they occurred only a couple times a year, but more recently they had increased to every two weeks. The severity of the pain depended on the climate, his emotions and the quality of sleep. The pain was fixed at the left temple. He had been given compound aminopyrine phenacetin tablets to stop the acute pain. His facial expression was flat, his tongue purple, and the pulse was deep and rough. The pattern was classified as blood stagnation affecting the collaterals. Treatment called for promoting blood movement to free stagnant blood. The prescription was House of Blood Stasis-Expelling Decoction. The formula included medicinals such as chuanxiong, bupleurum, carthamus, and others to promote the movement of qi and blood. He was told to cook one dose per day in water. After five doses, the intensity and frequency of the headaches had reduced. Twenty doses later, the headaches no longer occured. A two year follow-up reported that Mr. Chen was still without headaches and he had taken no further medication.

Case 3 - Migraine due to deficiency of qi and stagnant blood

Mrs. Li was 36 years old. Her first visit was in May 2001. She had experienced periodic episodes of migraines for more than twenty years. After trying a combined approach using Chinese medicine and biomedicine, she still suffered. Earlier treatments involved eliminating wind, calming the liver, promoting blood flow, expelling parasites and relieving pain. But the headaches were not relieved, and in fact continued to get worse. Her facial expression was pale, breath was short, she sweated under the slightest exertion, felt fatigued, and had a pale, dusky tongue. The patterns in Mrs. Li's case were deficiency of qi and stagnant blood. The treatment called for reinforcing qi and promoting blood flow in the channels. She was given a medicinal formula, which she cooked for herself every day. After 40 doses, the frequency of the headaches had decreased until they were finally eliminated. Several years have passed now without a relapse.

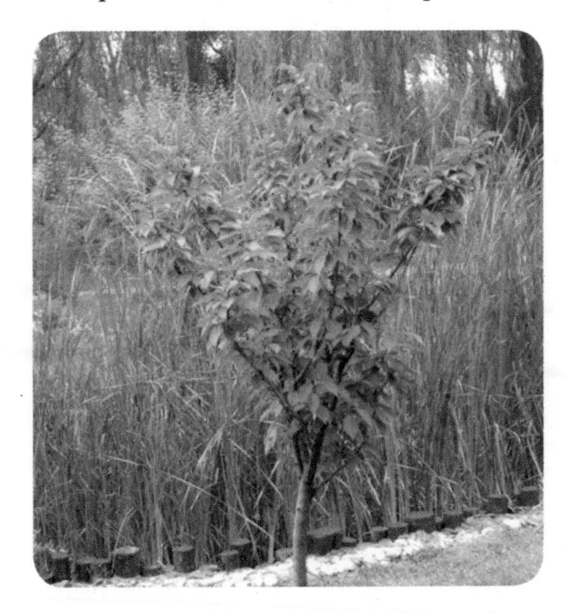

Case 4 - Acupuncture

Mrs. Guo was 23 years old when she first visited the clinic in March 2000. She had a history of migraines for which the prescription drug compound aminopyrine phenacetin usually worked. But recently her headaches had been more painful than normal and the medication only relieved the pain for one hour. Mrs. Guo decided to visit a Chinese medical clinic one morning. The headache was situated in her right eye socket. Her symptoms included throbbing pain in the right side of the head, especially in the right eye just below the center of the eyebrow at the point EX-HN4 (*yú yāo*). She supported her head with her hand, and did not want to open her eyes. Other symptoms included facial flushing, a runny nose, tearing of the eyes, and a tongue that was red at the tip and both sides. The practitioner determined that her headaches were due to wind-fire in the liver channel.

It was decided that in this case, acupuncture should be used rather than Chinese medicinals. Several points on the head and neck were needled, including GB 20 (*fēng chí*) and EX-HN5 (*tài yáng*), as well as a point on the liver channel on the foot, LV 2 (*xíng jiān*), in order to remove heat from that channel. The painful spot just below EX-HN4 (*yú yāo*) and another tender point near the eye were also needled. The needles were retained for 40 minutes. After the needles were withdrawn, her headache was relieved more than half, and did not increase again after leaving the treatment. After seven treatments, most of her symptoms had disappeared. A two year follow-up showed no relapse in the headaches.

Case 5 - Tui na

Mrs. Shi, a 45 years old female, visited the clinic in May 2004. Her chief complaint was headaches and she also experienced discomfort of the neck and nape, an aching back and shoulder pain, all of which had bothered her for three years. When the migraines occurred, pain-killers were necessary. Just one week before this visit to the clinic, she had fallen suddenly while walking. When it happened she was able to stand up immediately, but a few minutes later she felt a painful spasm in the nape of her neck along with stiffness in the shoulder and back, plus pain at the base of the skull. She had taken pain-killers 4-5 times per day since then. Occasionally she felt nauseous and sometimes vomited, and also had ringing in the ears and visual disturbances.

Upon examination no sign of abnormal cervical curvature was noted, but both sides of the neck muscles were tense, along with tenderness adjacent to the mid-cervical vertebrae. She had decreased range of neck motion left to right. An x-ray confirmed some joint stenosis, excess bone growth and hyperplasia, but the disks were normal. Rheoencephalogram showed limited blood supply to the basal artery. The diagnosis was vertebral artery type of cervical spondylosis. A tui na treatment plan was formulated that employed pushing, rubbing, pointing, pressing and grasping manipulations to points on the neck and head.

After five visits, she felt fewer spasms of the neck and was completely pain free in the nape. She was also able to reduce the dosage of the pain-killer she had been taking. After ten treatments the headache and other symptoms had been relieved significantly and she had completely stopped taking pharmaceuticals. When turning her neck, the remnant symptoms were not serious. After twenty treatments, the headaches were totally absent, and all symptoms had disappeared. From then on, only when her neck was fatigued would a mild migraine occur. Mrs. Shi was happy that her problem was cured without the need for surgery or more drugs.

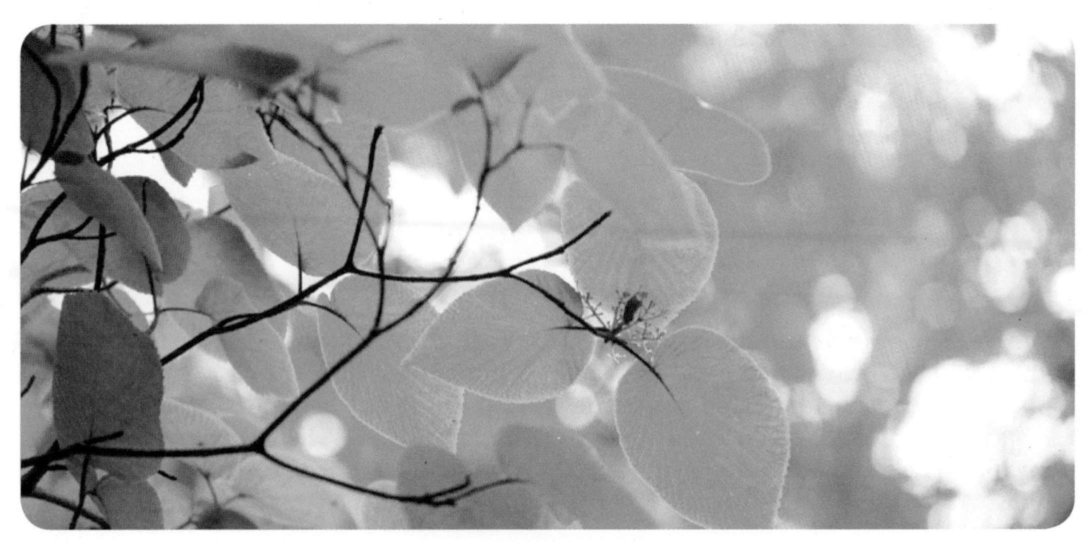

Conclusion

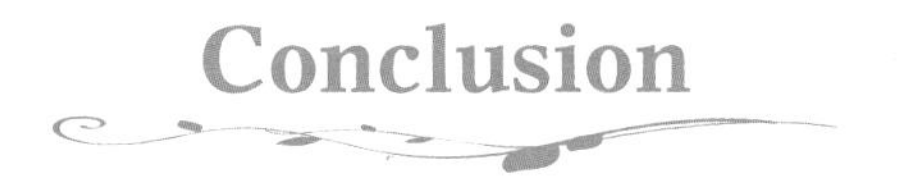

We hope this book has given you another option when it comes to managing your health.

Chinese medicine is not a magic pill, nor is biomedicine. Each system studies the amazing human body in its own way, with its own philosophy. Biomedicine sees the human body as a machine and analyzes each part in fantastic detail. Its strength is its precision and accuracy. Eventually, it will have the entire human body mapped out in the greatest detail. A doctor's job is to nail down the exact part that is broken down and fix it. As a patient, it is difficult to understand much about your treatments as biomedicine is extremely technical and there are so many details.

Meanwhile, Chinese medicine sketches a figure that is inseparable from his complex surroundings. In Chinese medicine, a person is neither a jigsaw puzzle nor a machine, but like a tree growing in soil, a fish swimming in water, or a bird flying in the sky. When it comes to accuracy and precision, Chinese medicine may never compare to biomedicine. Its strength is seeing the big picture. A practitioner's job is to evaluate the patient's general condition and find where the imbalances lie. As a patient, you may not have the training to evaluate your own imbalances of yin, yang, qi and blood, but you have the ability to understand what is wrong, and more importantly, how you can act to restore health.

In the future we think these two types of medicines will be integrated to benefit all mankind. It will take time. It will take understanding. Most of all, it will take wisdom, the wisdom to eliminate inhibition and choose freedom, the wisdom to judge by merit alone. Get the medicine you need, no matter Eastern or Western.

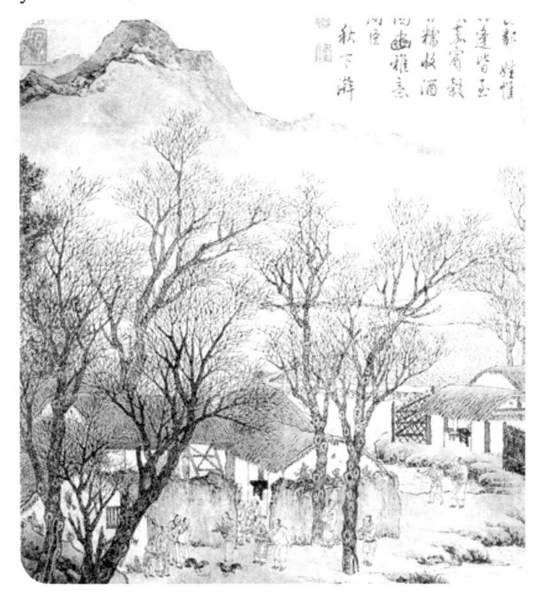

Appendix

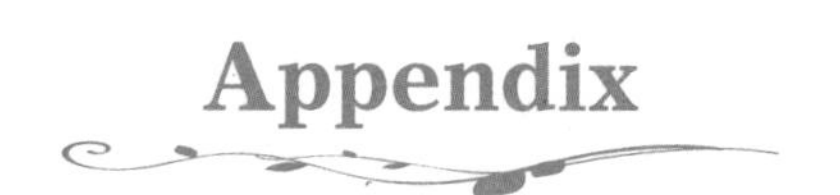

1. Additional Reading Material

Chinese medicine

- Xu Yi-bing. *An Illustrated Guide to Chinese Medicine.* People's Medical Publishing House, 2007
- Paul Pritchford. *Healing With Whole Foods: Asian Traditions and Modern Nutrition.* North Atlantic Books, 2003
- Harriet Beinfield, Efrem Korngold. *Between Heaven and Earth.* Random House, 1991
- Tom Williams. *Complete Illustrated Guide to Chinese Medicine.* Barnes & Noble INC, 1996
- http://www.acupuncture.com/education/tcmbasics/index.htm
- http://www.acupuncturetoday.com/abc/
- http://nccam.nih.gov/health/
- http://www.tcmstudent.com/
- http://www.nlm.nih.gov/hmd/chinese/chinesehome.html
- http://qi-journal.com/

Migraine headaches

- Oliver Sacks. *Migraine.* Vintage, 1999
- Diane Stafford, Jennifer Shoguist. *Migraines for Dummies.* For Dummies, 2003
- Lynn Constantine, Suzanne Scott. *Migraine: The Complete Guide.* Delta, 1994

Migraine headaches and Chinese medicine

- http://www.calvindale.com/treatments/headache.html
- http://www.holisticnetwork.org/articles/article_266.html
- http://www.tcmpage.com/hpheadaches.html
- http://findarticles.com/p/articles/mi_m0ISW/is_258/ai_n8592721
- http://www.acumedic.com/onestophealth/migraine.htm

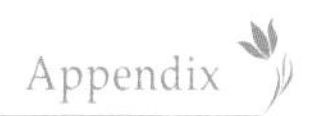

2. How to Find a Practitioner of Chinese Medicine ?

Finding a practitioner of Chinese medicine is often as easy as looking in your local phone book. Most cities now have an "Acupuncture" heading in the yellow pages. Since acupuncture is the most well known modality of Chinese medicine in Western countries, those that practice Chinese herbalism will also usually be listed in this section. In many places, there may not be a practitioner who specializes in treating migraines, but you may be able to find someone in the larger cities if you call around.

Most countries have established educational and licensure standards. A practitioner should be able to verify that these standards have been met.

The web can offer many ways to find a practitioner. Just searching for "acupuncture" and your town/area's name will probably locate something. The following internet resources should help you find a practitioner in your local area:

International Acupuncture Referral	http://www.acufinder.com http://www.gancao.net
Australia	Australian Acupuncture and Chinese Medicine Association http://www.acupuncture.org.au/
Canada	Traditional Chinese Medicine Association of British Columbia http://tcmabc.org/ Ordre des Acupuncteurs, Quebec http://www.ordredesacupuncteurs.qc.ca/
New Zealand	New Zealand Registrar of Acupuncture http://acupuncture.org.nz/
United Kingdom	Register of Chinese Herbal Medicine http://www.rchm.cwww.acupuncture.org.uk/ The British Medical Acupuncture Society http://www.medical-acupuncture.co.uk/
United States of America	National Certification Commission for Acupuncture and Oriental Medicine http://nccaom.org/ Council of Colleges of Acupuncture and Oriental Medicine http://www.ccaom.org/
Tai Ji – Qi Gong Information	http://www.worldtaichiday.org http://www.qi.org

References

1. Springhouse. *Professional Guide to Diseases (Eighth Edition)*. Lippincott Williams & Wilkins, 2005

2. The Development of Chinese Medicine. *http://www.bchg.org.cn/report/2007-04/1175780796d22.html*, 2007

3. National Institute of Health. Estimates of Funding for various Diseases, Conditions, Research Areas. *http://www.nih.gov/news/fundingresearchareas.htm*. 2007

4. Snow V, Weiss K, Wall EM, et al. Pharmacologic management of acute attacks of migraine headaches and prevention of migraine headache. *J. Ann Intern Med*. 2002, 137:840-849

5. Mathew NT. Dosing and administration of ergotamine tartrate and dihydroergotamine *Journal of Headaches*. 1997, 37(1):26-32

6. Bussone G, Manzoni GC, Cortelli P, et al. Efficacy and tolerability ofsumatriptan in the treatment of multiple migraine headaches attacks. *Journal of Neurological Science*. 2000, 21(2):272-278

7. Boureau F, Kappos L, Schoenen J, et al. A clinical comparison of sumatriptan nasal spray and dihydroergotamine nasal spray in the acute treatment of migraine headaches. *International Journal of Clinical Practice*. 2000 , 54(2):281-286

8. Spierings EL, Gomez MB, Grosz DE, et al. Oralalmotriptan vs oral sumatriptan in the abortive treatment of migraine headaches. *J. Arch Neurol*. 2001, 58(5):944-950

9. Gallagher RM, Dennish G, Spierings EL, et al. A comparative trial of zolmitriptan and sumatriptan for the acute oral treatment of migraine headaches. *Journal of Headache*. 2000, 40(1):119-128

10. Goadsby PJ, Ferrari MD, Olesen J, et al. Eletriptan in acute migraine headaches: a double-blind, placebo-controlled comparison to sumatriptan. *Journal of Neurology*. 2000, 54(1):156-163

11. Zhen C. The Pandemic of Influenza Eighty Years Ago. *Chinese Journal of Medical History*. No.4 1998

12. Molly Billings. The Influenza Pandemic of 1918. *http://virus.stanford.edu/uda/*, 1997

13. The Headache May Be Related to Diet. *http://www.people.com.cn/GB/channel2/570/20000926/251082.html*, 2000

14. Taylor-Piliae R, Haskell W, Stotts N, Froelicher E. Improvement in balance, strength, and flexibility after 12 weeks of tai ji in ethnic Chinese adults with cardiovascular disease risk factors. *Alternative Therapy Health Medicine*. 2006; 12(2):50-8.

15. Wannamethee G, Sharper A. Physical activity and strokes in British middle aged men. *British Medical Journal*. 1992; 304(6827), 597-601

16. Uusitupa M, Louheranta A, Lindstrom J, Valle T, Sundvall J, Eriksson J, Tuomilehto J. The Finnish diabetes prevention study. *British Journal of Nutrition*. 2000; 83(1),137-142

17. Hu Zhi-hui, Luo Dan. The Research of Relieve Pain with Laser Acupuncture. *Chinese Acupuncture& Moxibustion*. 2006; 26(7):533-534

18. Ted J Kapchuk. *The Web that Has No Weaver*. Contemporary Books, 2000

19. Ce J (Author), Li P (Translator), Li G (Translator), *Practical Chinese Qigong for Home Health Care*. Foreign Language Press, 1996

20. Omura, Y. Storing of qi gong energy in various materials and drugs (Qi Gongnization). *Acupuncture Electrotherapy Research*. 1990, 15(2):137-157

21. Wang Y. 65 kinds of pain treated with qi gong. *Chinese Qigong Science*. 1995, 2(6):39

22. Xu Yong-liang. Treat migraine headaches with qi gong to attack a vital point 35 cases. *Chinese Manipulation & Qi Gong Therapy*. 1996; (3):42

23. Shi Ling, Chen Jian. Treat the Low Back Pain Due to Stagnation of Liver Qi with Acupuncture. *Chinese Private Treatment*. 2003; 11(9):10-11

24. Wang Pai, Wu Yong-li, Zhang Yue-quan. The Observation of Acupuncture Treat Biliary Tract Pain. *Shanghai Journal of Acupuncture and Moxibustion*. 2003; 22(2):16-17

25. Tian K. *Acupuncture Treatment for Pain Symptoms.* Chinese Ancient Book Publishing Company. 2003, 3:172

26. Wu Y, Fang J. Intervening effect of different frequency electrostimulation on neuralgia. *Shanghai Journal of Acupuncture and Moxibustion.* 2007, 26(5):47-48

27.Du X. Experiences in the treatment of 40 cases of lateral head pain with matrix acupuncture-moxibustion. *Gansu Journal of Chinese Medicine.* 2003; 9:27-28

28. Zhou Jian-wei; Li Ji; Li Ning; Zhang Fan; Hu Ling-xiang; Zhao Jing-jing; Zhang Yan; Wang Cheng-wei. Transient Analgesic Effect of Electroacupuncture at Taiyang (EX-HN 5) for Treatment of Migraine headaches with Hyperactivity of the Liver-yang. *Chinese Acupuncture & Moxibustion.* 2007; 27(3):159-163

29. Li Gui-min; Ye De-bao. Research on the Effect of Electro-acupuncture of Neiguan on the CGRP Content in Migraine headaches Rats' Plasma. *Journal of Zhejiang University of Traditional Chinese Medicine.* 2007; 31(1):46-47

30. Zhang Shu-yan, Ma Ze-yun, Jin Guo-li. The Therapeutic and Effective Observation of Twisting and Shaking the Needle of Inserting to the Abutting Points in Order to Alleviate the Pain Felt During the Acute Stage of a Migraine headaches of a Blood Stasis Type. *Chinese Archives of Traditional Chinese Medicine.* 2007; 25(2):401-403

31. Yang Li-juan, Wu Yan, Li Bin. Treatment of Migraine headaches with Electroacupuncture and Auricular Acupoint Press Therapy. *Journal of Beijing University of Traditional Chinese Medicine(Clinical Medicine).* 2006; 13(5):26-27

32. Shen Yi-hua. Observations on the Efficacy of Electroacupuncture Plus Blood-letting Puncture for Treating Migraine headaches. *Shanghai Journal of Acupuncture and Moxibustion.* 2006; 25(9):15-16

33. Wang Bin. Nape Multiple Acupuncture Plus Surrounding Acupuncture for Migraine. *Shanghai Journal of Acupuncture and Moxibustion.* 2004; 23(4):14-15

34. Feng Shu-lan, He Xin-fang, Li Su-he. Clinical Observation of Migraine headaches by the Temporal Three Acupoints. *Journal of Clinical Acupuncture and Moxibustion.* 2003; 19(7):23-24

35. Liu Xian-liang, Tian Xiao-liang, Fan Chen-gen, Ji Gui-ying, Yang Guo-biao, Zhang Wei, Hu Xia. Clinical Study Report on Ordinary Ucgraine Treated by Acupuncture and Absorbing O_2. *Journal of Clinical Medical Officer.* 2002; 30(2):47-48

36. Zhang Da-jun. Treat Migraine headaches Due to Excessive Rising of Liver-yang with Tian Ma Gou Teng Yin. *Chinese Journal of Modern Chinese and Western Medicine.* 2007; 5(8):25

37. Xu Jian-ping, Zheng Jian-peng. Treat Migraine headaches 104 Cases with Tao Hong Si Wu Tang. *Journal of Practical Traditional Chinese Internal Medicine.* 2004; (5):35

38. Li Yong-hua. Treat Migraine headaches Due to Blood Stasis with Tong Qiao Huo Xue Tang. *Chinese Community Doctors.* 2005; (16):40

39. Hu HQ, Zhou YH, Wang XL. Clinical Study on Effect of Xiaoyao Nose Drops in Stopping Episode of Migraine headaches. *Chinese Journal of Integrative Medicine.* 2006; 12(2):112

40. Hu ZQ, Song LG, Mei T. Clinical and Experimental Study on Treatment of Migraine headaches with shutianning Granule. *Chinese Journal of Integrated Traditional and Western Medicine.* 2002; 22(8):581

41. Di Shu-qing, Di Li-wei, Liu Cui-xin. Treat 46 cases of migraine headaches with Quan Tian Ma Capsule. *Chinese Journal of Misdiagnosis.* 2007; (24):30

42. Zhong Lian-jiang, Zhang Ning-yuan. Treat 36 cases of migraine headaches with San Chong Ding Tong Decoction. *Journal of Practical Traditional Chinese Internal Medicine.* 2007; (5):22

43. Huang Ning, Chen Zhi-lin, Li Chen-dong. Treat 37 cases of migraine headaches with Modified Chai Hu Long Gu Mu Li Decoction. *Jiangsu Journal of Traditional Chinese Medicine.* 2007; (11):14

44. Zhang Jin-mei. Treat 105 cases of migraine headaches with clearing heat, calming the liver and eliminating wind to stop pain. *Journal of Emergency in Traditional Chinese Medicine.* 2007; (9):54

45. Xu He-xian. The clinical curative effect observation of Man Jing Zi Tou Feng Decoction to treat migraine headaches. *Medical Journal of Chinese People's Health.* 2007; (20):36

46. Zhu De-cai, Xiang Fu-sheng. *Massage and Daoyin,* 2003(2).

47. Wang Zhen, Zhou Xiao-yan, Yao Le. A case report of migraine patient cured by massage. *Massage and Daoyin,* 2003(5).

48. Meng Bo-ping, Meng Hai-bin and Chen Lin. The clinical application and theoretical discussion of massage in treating migraine of cervical origin. *Massage and Daoyin,* 2003(6).

Index

T

U

V

W

X

Y

Z

图书在版编目（CIP）数据

中医科普系列——偏头痛（英文）/王蕾等主编. —北京：
人民卫生出版社，2008. 10
ISBN 978 - 7 - 117 - 10505 - 7

Ⅰ. 中… Ⅱ. 王… Ⅲ. 偏头痛 - 中医治疗法 - 英文
Ⅳ. R277. 772

中国版本图书馆 CIP 数据核字（2008）第 119371 号

中医科普系列——偏头痛
（英文）

主　　编：王　蕾　卡尔·斯蒂姆森
出版发行：人民卫生出版社（中继线 +8610 - 6761 - 6688）
地　　址：中国北京丰台区方庄芳群园三区 3 号楼
邮　　编：100078
网　　址：http：//www. pmph. com
E - mail：pmphsales@ gmail. com
购书热线：+8610 - 6769 - 1034（电话及传真）
开　　本：850 × 1168　1/24
版　　次：2008 年 10 月第 1 版　2008 年 10 月第 1 版第 1 次印刷
标准书号：ISBN 978 - 7 - 117 - 10505 - 7/R · 10506